By The Editors of Consumer Guide®

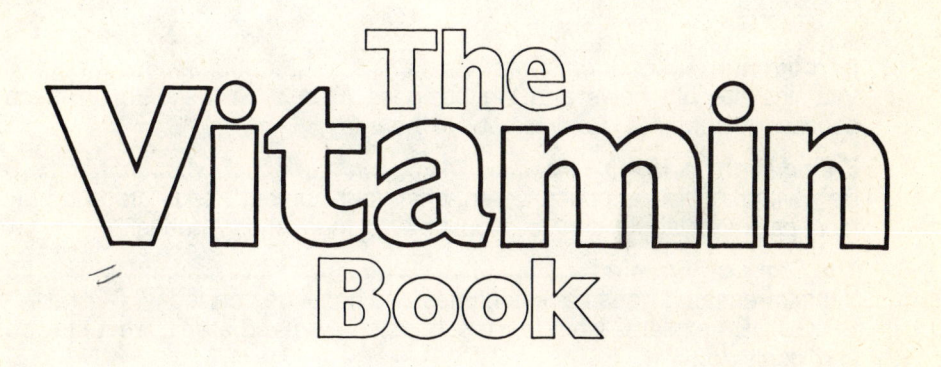

The Vitamin Book

Copyright© 1979 by Publications International, Ltd.
All rights reserved
This book may not be reproduced or quoted in whole or in part by mimeograph or any other printed means or for presentation on radio or television without written permission from:

Louis Weber, President
Publications International Ltd.
3841 West Oakton Street
Skokie, Illinois 60076

Permission is never granted for commercial purposes.

Manufactured in the United States of America
1 2 3 4 5 6 7 8 9 10

LIBRARY OF CONGRESS CATALOG
CARD NUMBER: 79-89737

ISBN: 0-671-25199-6 (cloth)
　　　　0-671-24819-7

Consulting Editors
Terry Alan Sandholzer
Karen M. Sandrick
Cover Photo
Dave Jordano Photography Inc.
Cover Design
Frank E. Peiler

Contents

Introduction...4
Vitamins are big news and big business. Here's all the data on these necessary nutrients, from history to hearsay.

Eating Right Is Up to You..8
Be a vitamin-wise shopper. Learn what your nutrient needs are and how food package labels can tell you how to meet those needs.

The Story of Vitamins...25
Vitamin research goes back centuries and continues on today. CONSUMER GUIDE® explains what these substances are and aren't; what they do and don't do.

Thiamin (Vitamin B_1)...39
A source of instant energy? A fatigue fighter and appetite booster?

Riboflavin (Vitamin B_2).......................................52
Essential to the body's generation of energy, riboflavin has been claimed to play a role in preventing cataracts. See what the experts say.

Niacin...64
Prevent heart attacks with a vitamin? Large doses of niacin can reduce cholesterol in the blood, but our experts urge caution.

Pantothenic Acid..78
Some animal studies indicate that this vitamin can help prevent gray hair and even arthritis; but there's no proof that humans can derive such benefits.

Vitamin B_6 (Pyridoxine).......................................86
Ease morning sickness? Relieve migraines?

Biotin...96
Despite claims to the effect that biotin deficiency can lead to heart attacks and mental disorders, our experts found no reason for most people to boost biotin intake.

Folacin...102
Are you pregnant, breast-feeding, or taking oral contraceptives? If so, then you may need more folacin than others. But our experts found that there's more than enough folacin for anyone right in a healthy diet.

Vitamin B$_{12}$ (Cyanocobalamin) 111
Claimed to be the "antianemia vitamin," B$_{12}$ plays an important role in cell formation; but there's no evidence to support its supposed "energy-boosting" capabilities.

Vitamin C (Ascorbic Acid) 120
Nobel Prize winner Linus Pauling has convinced millions that C is effective in preventing and curing the common cold. But what do the controlled studies show?

Vitamin A (Retinol) 138
The "carrot vitamin," A plays an important role in preventing night blindness. Excessive doses, however, can be toxic.

Vitamin D 152
Necessary for strong teeth and bones, vitamin D is claimed to be effective in preventing arthritis and myopia. But the evidence points to more hazard than benefit in consuming excess amounts.

Vitamin E (Tocopherol) 160
Prevent heart attacks? Slow the aging process? Enhance sexual potency? The true believers make such claims for vitamin E, but controversy rages. Here are the facts as they stand today.

Vitamin K 170
Caution! Excessive intake of one form of vitamin K can be hazardous. Our experts tell you how much you need and how to get it.

Vitamin Supplements 175
Vitamin supplements are *not* substitutes for eating a good diet. They may be necessary in special cases, but do you really need them?

Megavitamin Therapy 192
If some is good, is mega better? Our experts diagnose the promise and pitfalls of taking massive doses.

Minerals 198
Minerals are the nutrient companions of vitamins.

Vitamin Supplement Profiles 219
If you're determined to invest in "nutrition insurance," here are evaluative profiles of nearly 70 brand-name vitamin supplements.

Glossary 263

Bibliography 270

Suggested Reading 272

References 273

Index 279

Introduction

The sailors were dying. After weeks at sea, symptoms developed among ships' crews that must have reminded some of the dreaded plagues on land. Men became weak. Their skin discolored. Their gums bled, and their teeth fell out. A surgeon on one of His Majesty's ships followed a hunch. He suspected that it was something the men weren't getting in their food that caused their sickness and that the cure lay in the simple addition of that "something" to the daily diet.

The ailment was scurvy. The missing substance was the "magic" nutrient in citrus fruits, vitamin C. With the requisition of lime juice for all sailors, scurvy ceased being the scourge of the British navy.

Introduction

The history of vitamins reads like a mystery story with a scientific bent. Once, no one even knew vitamins were there. People ate food for centuries without caring about what was in it. Eventually, curious scientists began to investigate why the deprivation of certain "unknowns" made people sick. Today, after years of studies and experiments, the keys to good health seem to have been found. And one of those keys is vitamins.

Now that it is known that vitamins exist and are important, everyone wants to know all about them. Articles about vitamins and vitamin supplements appear regularly in popular magazines, and scores of books about vitamins are gobbled up by the reading public every year.

Such curiosity would have been satisfied long ago if all the stories told were consistent and accurate. But each new publication seems to promote new ideas and make new claims for one particular vitamin or another—claims that find an eager audience and offer hope of cures that, many times, cannot be substantiated.

After a time and many claims later, it's hard to tell who said what about a particular vitamin and whether what was said was based on fact or on fantasy. Certainly, if all the claims were true, our national health would be optimum, but it isn't. A look at what has been said about vitamin E will cast light on the confusion.

In the last decade or so, vitamin E has been recommended by one source or another for the cure or prevention of heart disease, acne, liver spots, muscular dystrophy, sterility, sexual impotency and some fifty more maladies. Yet, none of these claims is true. And if you're buying and using a vitamin E supplement to cure or prevent any of these conditions, you're wasting your money and perhaps endangering your life.

Where did these claims about vitamins come from? Who started them? And why have they continued to be believed by a large portion of the public?

There's no doubt that vitamins are essential for good health. Each vitamin has a function to perform in the

Introduction

human body. But what happens if you take more than you need? If you take a vitamin supplement will you be doing yourself any good? Any harm? Will you be spending money needlessly? What are vitamins, anyway?

CONSUMER GUIDE® magazine, working with recognized experts in the fields of medicine and nutrition, has uncovered the unusual histories of these essential nutrients called vitamins. We have cut through the confusion and have come up with a clear understanding about each vitamin's function, value, and the dangers of deficiency and overdose. We cite the sources of each vitamin and provide you with menus to help you get the vitamins you need, naturally, through the foods you eat.

To clear up the controversy, we list the most famous claims made for each vitamin and discuss their merits, their shortcomings, and, in some cases, their dangers. A chapter on minerals highlights those important nutrients and how they function in the human body. We report on the research that is currently going on in the field of nutritional science. And we inform you of governmental regulations concerning the manufacture and sale of vitamins—regulations that affect millions of people in this country.

Throughout this book, we emphasize that proper diet and an adherence to the recommended intake of each vitamin (as established by governmental boards and panels) will supply you with all the vitamins your body needs for good health. If, after all this, you're still looking for that elusive "vitamin insurance" through vitamin supplements, we provide clear-cut instructions on how to read the labels of over-the-counter preparations and offer information to help you decide whether or not you need extra vitamins. We tell you what supplements you should and should not buy, profiling and commenting on over 65 multivitamin and multivitamin-plus-mineral products. (A separate chapter on megavitamin therapy discusses the dangerous trend toward self-diagnosis and self-treatment of nonexistent vitamin deficiencies with large doses of vitamin supplements and the use of massive doses to

Introduction

prevent and cure a variety of physical and mental diseases.)

When you've finished this book, we hope you will be an acting "expert" on vitamins, one who is more aware of what you *do* eat and what you *should* eat. We hope that this information compels you to select food consciously to keep your nutritional edge sharp. The following chapters build up from basic nutrition and show how all its elements fit together. Enjoy your reading, your eating, and here's to your good health.

Eating Right Is Up to You

Studying only vitamins in the school of nutrition is like only studying verbs in an English class. To know how vitamins work, you also must know how they relate to one another and where they fit among the elements of basic nutrition. In understanding what food contains, why we need it, and how it's used in our bodies, we can more fully understand the sometimes intricate workings of foods' all-vital vitamins. And with this knowledge, we have it within our power to eat better and be healthy.

Nutrition can be defined as the sum of the processes by which an animal or plant absorbs and utilizes food substances. An understanding of nutrition requires

Eating Right Is Up to You

knowledge of food composition, the digestive processes, and body chemistry or metabolism. It's also important to understand why people eat as they do—the economic, religious, ethnic, and social factors which influence food choices.

History

People have walked the face of the earth for 250,000 years. For most of that time they were hunters and gatherers, scrounging for food among the plants and killing the animals in their territories to nourish themselves and to go on living. When food sources became scarce, tribes and individuals moved on to greener pastures . . . or perished.

About 10,000 years ago, human beings developed agriculture. They began to farm and to domesticate animals, thereby working with the environment to take care of themselves. From ignorance evolved curiosity about how food sustains life. With the dawning of the scientific age, people began to ask questions about what happens to the food that is eaten, about how food generates energy, and about what foods are important for growth and for maintaining life itself. These and other questions could not be answered until chemistry, biochemistry, physiology, and other related sciences had advanced.

In the late 1700s, Antoine Lavoisier, a Frenchman often considered the "Father of Nutrition," investigated the relationships between respiration and energy production. His studies showed that the oxygen in the air we inhale is used up as body heat and energy is produced. He also observed that, in the process, carbon dioxide is created and exhaled. Lavoisier concluded that food is the fuel which is oxidized or "burned up" in the body to produce and release energy. This body process has been described as a "slow furnace." In a coal furnace, for example, coal burns in the presence of oxygen and releases carbon dioxide and energy in the form of heat. The oxidation of

Eating Right Is Up to You

food is a similar process, but we know now that oxidation is a complex and carefully controlled body function. Lavoisier's work was the first step to uncovering how food is used to sustain life. The process to that end is called metabolism.

Metabolism and Energy

Metabolism applies to all the chemical reactions which take place in the body and within each of the body's billions of cells. These chemical reactions are necessary for the production of hundreds of compounds which are vital to the process of life. The proteins of muscles, the hormones, and the fats are examples of such necessary compounds. Metabolism also involves chemical and physical reactions which help rid the body of substances it no longer needs. The process of using food as fuel is referred to as *energy metabolism.*

Energy is simply the ability to do work. Today, we talk about the energy value of foods and about the number of calories in a particular food. The calorie is a unit of heat energy; that is, it measures energy as a form of heat. The energy value of individual foods depends on the amount of carbohydrates, fats, and proteins present. Measured in calories per gram, carbohydrates and proteins supply four calories per gram, and fats yield nine calories per gram. (One gram is often described as equal to the weight of a paper clip. There are 28.3 grams in an ounce and 454 grams in a pound. A milligram is one-thousandth of a gram; a microgram is one-millionth of a gram, or one-thousandth of a milligram.)

Different types of energy are interchangeable. For example, the chemical energy of carbohydrates, which are important body fuels, can be converted to heat energy to help maintain a constant body temperature. It also can be changed to kinetic energy necessary for muscle action and physical activity or trapped as chemical energy in other body compounds.

Eating Right Is Up to You

The Essential Nutrients

As chemistry developed in the 18th and 19th centuries, so did procedures to analyze what we eat. Scientists soon discovered the great variety of chemically distinct compounds in foods. Ongoing experiments determined what foods and what parts of foods are best suited for growth and health.

In 1827 the English physician William Prout described the three "staminal principles" of foods necessary to support life: the oily, the saccharin and the albuminous principles. These are recognized today as fats (and oils), carbohydrates, and proteins. Believing that a diet which supplies these substances would be nutritionally satisfactory, Prout was probably the first to define an "adequate diet."

The study of food chemistry became increasingly sophisticated. Researchers began to use animals in their investigations. By the latter part of the 19th century, the "adequate diet" proposed by Prout was expanded to include minerals or inorganic elements. Today, at least sixteen inorganic elements are recognized as essential nutrients for man.

Then at the opening of this century, a fifth class of nutrients was uncovered. Scientists found that experimental animals perished if they were fed diets containing only highly purified preparations of fat, carbohydrate, protein, and the known inorganic elements. The missing vital nutrients turned out to be vitamins. (Earlier workers had failed to recognize the existence of vitamins because the diets prepared for experimental animals were not sufficiently "pure"; they were "contaminated" with vitamins.) Thirteen necessary vitamins now are known. The last, vitamin B_{12}, was discovered in the 1940s. An adequate diet is described as one that supplies all of these essential nutrients in appropriate amounts and, at the same time, does not contribute too much of those nutrients which are potentially harmful if taken in excess.

Eating Right Is Up to You

The first table at the end of this chapter briefly describes the nature and function of the five classes of essential nutrients.

Recommended Dietary Allowances

Requirements for the essential nutrients vary from person to person and with age, sex, physiological state (e.g., pregnancy), and physical activity. Even among people of the same age, sex, and life-style, essential nutrient needs are not precisely the same. To develop a list which would precisely describe every individual's requirements is impossible.

However, there are standards—known as the Recommended Dietary Allowances (RDAs)—which have been established by the Food and Nutrition Board of the National Academy of Sciences, National Research Council. They provide general guidelines to be followed to get the nutrients needed for good health. The first RDA table was published in 1943 during World War II, an outgrowth of the need to determine the food and nutrition situation in the United States as it related to national defense. The productivity of the American people was dependent upon good health, and good health depended upon good nutrition.

The first list contained the recommended daily intake for calories, protein, six vitamins and two inorganic elements. To encompass new findings in the nutrition field, the list has grown until, as of 1974, the RDA incorporates 10 vitamins and six inorganic elements. As yet, there are no RDAs for three of the 13 vitamins and for many of the essential inorganic elements. But research goes on. New nutrients may yet be discovered.

RDAs are not minimum dietary requirements. They represent the amounts of nutrients which will meet the needs of all normal, healthy people. With the exception of allowances for calories, the RDAs contain a "margin of safety": They are deliberately set at levels higher than

Eating Right Is Up to You

estimated for the average person. This margin of safety allows for individual requirements and for those occasional but inevitable stress situations which occur in everyday life. (RDAs are not intended to and cannot serve as guidelines for the nutritional management of seriously ill persons or of those with genetic or metabolic disorders that cause profound changes in nutrient needs.)

Failure to strictly follow the RDAs in the diet will not automatically cause deficiencies, however. The RDAs are optimum figures which, if attained, will provide the best possible nutrition. If your diet supplies the recommended amounts of all nutrients for which RDAs have been established, the needs for those nutrients not included in the RDA table also will be met.

The RDAs have been criticized because they have fluctuated over the 30-year period since their establishment and because they differ from the nutrient standards of other countries and those of international health organizations. But this fluctuation should be considered as growth, not indecision by those who work to maintain the appropriateness of the RDAs. The RDAs change to reflect new scientific data that come to light.

Other dietary standards have often been established with goals and philosophies different from those of the Food and Nutrition Board. Some are set at levels designed to prevent deficiencies, but not necessarily to provide optimal intakes for all people.

The latest Table of Recommended Dietary Allowances is reproduced at the end of this chapter. (See pages 21 to 23.) It reflects 17 different age-sex categories. The individual vitamin chapters which follow indicate the RDAs for adult men and women where they have been established. You may refer back to this table for information about the RDAs for infants, children, and teenagers.

The "Basic Four" Food Groups

To help people plan and evaluate their diets for adequate

Eating Right Is Up to You

nutrition, the United States Department of Agriculture developed the "Daily Food Guide," an easily understood plan for selecting foods. (See the table below.) Commonly referred to as the "Basic Four" or the "Four Food Group Guide," this plan reflects the nutrient content and deficiency in each food group. Foods in the meat group—which includes nuts, dried beans and peas—are high in protein, for example, whereas fruits and vegetables contribute little protein. On the other hand, vegetables are a good source of many vitamins, some of which are present only in small

---

THE "BASIC FOUR" FOOD GROUP PLAN
A Recommended Daily Guide

Milk Group
2 servings/adults
4 servings/teenagers
3 servings/children
 Foods made from milk contribute part of the nutrients supplied by a serving of milk.

Meat Group
2 servings
 Dry beans and peas, soy extenders, and nuts combined with animal protein (meat, fish, poultry, eggs, milk, cheese) or grain protein can be substituted for a serving of meat.

Fruit-Vegetable Group
4 servings
 Dark green, leafy, or orange vegetables and fruit are recommended three or four times weekly. Citrus fruit is recommended daily.

Cereal Group
4 servings
 Whole-grain, fortified, or enriched grain products are recommended.

Others
 Fats, oils, and sweets complement but do not replace foods from the "Basic Four" groups. Amounts should be determined by individual caloric needs.

Eating Right Is Up to You

amounts in meats. Milk and milk products are excellent sources of calcium, an essential nutrient not provided in any significant amount by meats or cereals.

Daily diets which include the recommended number of servings from each of the four food groups will supply adequate amounts of the essential nutrients (with the possible exception of iron). The total amount of necessary calories depends upon an individual's age, sex, physical activity, and general health.

Teenage girls and women in their childbearing years have trouble meeting the RDA for iron with usual diets because they need a relatively large amount of this trace element to replace what is lost during menstruation. Iron-rich foods, such as liver and foods fortified with iron, should be eaten frequently. Physicians and nutritionists often recommend the use of iron supplements by girls and women to ensure an adequate intake.

A diet with only the minimum number of servings suggested by the Four Food Group plan furnishes about 1,200 calories—a good diet goal for persons trying to lose weight. Physically active people and young people who are still growing need more than 1,200 calories and should add more foods to the core diet to get those extra calories. Or foods included in the "fifth group" can be added. Here we find fats and oils (butter, margarine, salad dressings) and sweets (sugar, candy, rich desserts). These are not included in any of the basic four groups because they have what nutritionists call a "low nutrient density" (popularly referred to as "empty calories"). They supply calories but they contribute little or no protein, vitamins, or inorganic elements to the diet.

Further, not all the foods in any one of the four groups have the same nutritional value. For example, some foods in the fruit and vegetable group are much better sources of vitamin C or vitamin A than are others. So the selection made to meet the daily recommendations for each group will affect the overall nutrient content of the diet.

Even though a diet fulfills the recommendations of the

Eating Right Is Up to You

Daily Food Guide, there is no guarantee that the RDAs for all nutrients will be furnished. Variety is the key. Only by varying the choices from each group from day to day will you be assured of getting the necessary nutrients.

The Four Food Group plan is not without its critics. Some argue that among the thousands of foods available there are many which do not fit well into any single group. Where does pizza belong, for example? With its sausage, cheese, tomato sauce, and crust, all four food groups are represented.

Dietary recommendations based on serving size may also be confusing. Certainly the quantity is not the same for all people. Although a serving of meat is usually considered as three ounces, this portion may be too much for some, too little for others.

The suggestion to eat a variety of foods from different classes may seem like an overly simplistic approach. But simplicity may make it easier to remember what to eat, and if it's easier we're more likely to do it. Foods of similar nutritional value are grouped together, and each group has its own unique part to play in contributing the required nutrients. The Basic Four Plan is a useful guide to good nutrition. You can select the foods you enjoy from each group, and the variety makes it possible for you to avoid the things you do not like.

Product Labeling

In response to the growing consumer interest in food values, the federal government instituted a means by which all consumer food goods can be labeled. The "Nutrition Information" panels on canned, frozen and boxed goods help consumers to become familiar with nutrient terminology and guide them toward an intake of adequate amounts of the established essential nutrients.

The nutrient values are listed as "United States Recommended Daily Allowances (U.S. RDAs). Although based on the Recommended Dietary Allowances from the Food

Eating Right Is Up to You

and Nutrition Board, they are not the same. The U.S. RDA for a specific nutrient is usually the highest value for that nutrient (currently based on the 1968 RDA table and excluding pregnant and lactating women). The third table at the end of this chapter (page 24) shows the U.S. RDAs which are used for the nutrition information panel on most foods. (Other U.S. RDA lists have been established for the labeling of foods specifically designed for infants, children under 4 years of age, and for pregnant and lactating women.)

FDA regulations require that the nutrition information panel be included on labels of all enriched or fortified foods. The information panel is also mandatory if any claim for nutritional quality is made elsewhere on the label or in advertisements for the food. Even when the panel is included voluntarily by the food manufacturer, information must be provided in terms of the U.S. RDAs for protein, five vitamins and two inorganic elements. (Information about seven additional vitamins and four more inorganic elements is optional.)

A typical nutrition information panel is shown on the next page. The number of servings in the package or container and the size of a single serving are shown at the top as required. The amount of carbohydrate, fat, and protein (in grams) and the number of calories in a serving are given. Under certain circumstances this section may include the amount of sodium and cholesterol in a serving.

The quality of the food with respect to protein, vitamins, and inorganic elements is indicated under the heading "Percentage of U.S. Recommended Daily Allowances (U.S. RDA)." In the sample panel shown, one serving (two slices) of wheat bread contains, for example, 15 percent of the U.S. RDA for thiamin; 8 percent for iron; and 0 percent for vitamin C. Using these figures and the U.S. RDA values shown in the table on page 24, it is possible to calculate the actual amount of these nutrients present; 0.23 mg thiamin, 1.44 mg iron, and no vitamin C.

Even without going through the mathematics, consum-

Eating Right Is Up to You

SAMPLE OF NUTRITION INFORMATION PANEL
The sample panel below was taken from a loaf of wheat bread.

Nutrition Information per Serving		Percentage of U.S. Recommended Daily Allowances (U.S. RDA)	
Serving Size	2 ounces (approx. 2 slices)		Per 2 oz. Serving
Servings per pkg.	12		
Calories	150		
Protein	5 grams	Protein	8
Carbohydrates	26 grams	Vitamin A	0
Fat	3 grams	Vitamin C	0
Cholesterol*	below 5 milligrams	Thiamin	15
		Riboflavin	8
Less than 5 mg cholesterol per 100 grams		Niacin	10
		Calcium	6
		Iron	8

*Information on cholesterol is provided for individuals who, on the advice of a physician, are modifying their total dietary intake of cholesterol.

---

ers can use nutrition labeling to help them select foods. A high percentage of the U.S. RDA value for a nutrient suggests that the food is a good source of that nutrient. Conversely, a low or zero value indicates that the nutrient is not present in any significant amount. The panels then can be used to compare nutritional quality of similar foods. For example, a comparison will show that peaches are better sources of vitamin A than are pears, that orange juice has more vitamin C than apple juice.

In addition to health-conscious people, nutrition labeling aids calorie-counters as well. A food that contains a fairly high percentage of the U.S. RDA for several nutrients but

Eating Right Is Up to You

relatively few calories can assure dieters of getting their daily nutrient requirements while still controlling the calories.

Nutrition information is not yet available for all foods. It is currently confined to canned, bottled, or otherwise packaged foods, but federal agencies are exploring ways to extend the system to include fresh meats, fruits, and vegetables.

As a consumer who is sincerely interested in planning diets that are nutritionally sufficient, you can easily do so. The Daily Food Guide is a simple, easy-to-use plan. The introduction of nutrition labeling has made more detailed information about actual nutrient content of foods available.

This book focuses on one class of essential nutrients—vitamins. Included in the following chapters are discussions of each vitamin's function, its role in metabolism, signs and symptoms of deficiency and toxicity, its possible use for therapeutic purposes, and its food sources. It's important to note also that vitamins do not stand alone but relate to one another and to other essential nutrients. With a clear understanding of these vital elements of nutrition, you will have the ability to select the proper foods your body needs to live a healthier, happier life.

Eating Right Is Up to You

CLASSES OF ESSENTIAL NUTRIENTS

Nutrient Class	Major Functions
Carbohydrates Starches; Sugars	Used primarily to supply energy; carbohydrates furnish 4 calories per gram.
Fats and Oils (Lipids) Essential fatty acids	Used to supply energy; fats furnish 9 calories per gram. A layer of fat under the skin insulates the body. Fat around internal organs cushions and protects them. Accumulation of too much fat leads to overweight and obesity. Dietary fat supplies the "essential fatty acids," important components of cells. The body cannot synthesize them.
Proteins Essential amino acids	Primary function is growth and maintenance of muscle or lean body tissues. Proteins can be used for energy, furnishing 4 calories per gram. Proteins are made up of smaller units — the amino acids — eight of which are essential; they cannot be made by the body.
Vitamins	Function as regulators of body chemistry or metabolism. Necessary for normal synthesis and breakdown of body carbohydrates, fats, and proteins. Many play a role as coenzymes.
Inorganic Elements (Minerals)* Macroelements: calcium, chloride, magnesium, phosphorus, potassium, sodium Microelements (trace elements): chromium, cobalt, copper, fluorine, iodine, iron, manganese, molybdenum, selenium, zinc Water	As an important part of bones some elements (e.g., calcium and phosphorus) contribute to body structure. Iron is a part of hemoglobin, the red pigment in blood which transports oxygen from the lungs to the tissues. Inorganic elements in body fluids help in maintaining normal acid-base balance and in regulating water balance. Some inorganic elements are essential for normal responses of nerves and muscles to stimuli. Certain inorganic elements are important regulators of body chemistry and are essential for normal enzyme action. Water accounts for 60 percent of body weight. Water is a constituent of every cell in the body. Blood, a water solution, carries nutrients to cells and waste products from them.

See the chapter on minerals for complete details of the inorganic elements.

20

Eating Right Is Up to You

FOOD AND NUTRITION BOARD, NATIONAL ACADEMY OF SCIENCES-NATIONAL RESEARCH COUNCIL RECOMMENDED DAILY DIETARY ALLOWANCES,[a] **Revised 1974**

Designed for the maintenance of good nutrition of practically all healthy people in the U.S.A.

	Age (years)	Weight (kg)	Weight (lbs)	Height (cm)	Height (in)	Energy (kcal)[b]	Protein (g)	Vitamin A Activity (RE)[c]	(IU)	Vitamin D (IU)	Vitamin E Activity[e] (IU)
Infants	0.0-0.5	6	14	60	24	kg × 117	kg × 2.2	420[d]	1,400	400	4
	0.5-1.0	9	20	71	28	kg × 108	kg × 2.0	400	2,000	400	5
Children	1-3	13	28	86	34	1,300	23	400	2,000	400	7
	4-6	20	44	110	44	1,800	30	500	2,500	400	9
	7-10	30	66	135	54	2,400	36	700	3,500	400	10
Males	11-14	44	97	158	63	2,800	44	1,000	5,000	400	12
	15-18	61	134	172	69	3,000	54	1,000	5,000	400	15
	19-22	67	147	172	69	3,000	54	1,000	5,000	400	15
	23-50	70	154	172	69	2,700	56	1,000	5,000		15
	51+	70	154	172	69	2,400	56	1,000	5,000		15
Females	11-14	44	97	155	62	2,400	44	800	4,000	400	12
	15-18	54	119	162	65	2,100	48	800	4,000	400	12
	19-22	58	128	162	65	2,100	46	800	4,000	400	12
	23-50	58	128	162	65	2,000	46	800	4,000		12
	51+	58	128	162	65	1,800	46	800	4,000		12
Pregnant						+300	+30	1,000	5,000	400	15
Lactating						+500	+20	1,200	6,000	400	15

Fat-Soluble Vitamins

[a] The allowances are intended to provide for individual variations among most normal persons as they live in the United States under the usual environmental stresses. Diets should be based on a variety of common foods in order to provide other nutrients for which human requirements have been less well defined.
[b] Kilojoules (kJ) = 4.2 × kcal.
[c] Retinol equivalents.
[d] Assumed to be all as retinol in milk during the first six months of life. All subsequent intakes are assumed to be half as retinol and half as β-carotene when calculated from international units. As retinol equivalents, three fourths are as retinol and one fourth as β-carotene.
[e] Total vitamin E activity, estimated to be 80 percent as α-tocopherol and 20 percent other tocopherols.
(Published with permission.)

Eating Right Is Up to You

FOOD AND NUTRITION BOARD, NATIONAL ACADEMY OF SCIENCES-NATIONAL RESEARCH COUNCIL RECOMMENDED DAILY DIETARY ALLOWANCES,[a] Revised 1974 (CONTINUED)

	Age (years)	Weight (kg)	Weight (lbs)	Height (cm)	Height (in)	Energy (kcal)[b]	Protein (g)	Ascorbic Acid (mg)	Folacin[f] (μg)	Niacin[g] (mg)	Riboflavin (mg)	Thiamin (mg)	Vitamin B_6 (mg)	Vitamin B_{12} (μg)
Infants	0.0-0.5	6	14	60	24	kg X 117	kg X 2.2	35	50	5	0.4	0.3	0.3	0.3
	0.5-1.0	9	20	71	28	kg X 108	kg X 2.0	35	50	8	0.6	0.5	0.4	0.3
Children	1-3	13	28	86	34	1,300	23	40	100	9	0.8	0.7	0.6	1.0
	4-6	20	44	110	44	1,800	30	40	200	12	1.1	0.9	0.9	1.5
	7-10	30	66	135	54	2,400	36	40	300	16	1.2	1.2	1.2	2.0
Males	11-14	44	97	158	63	2,800	44	45	400	18	1.5	1.4	1.6	3.0
	15-18	61	134	172	69	3,000	54	45	400	20	1.8	1.5	2.0	3.0
	19-22	67	147	172	69	3,000	54	45	400	20	1.8	1.5	2.0	3.0
	23-50	70	154	172	69	2,700	56	45	400	18	1.6	1.4	2.0	3.0
	51+	70	154	172	69	2,400	56	45	400	16	1.5	1.2	2.0	3.0
Females	11-14	44	97	155	62	2,400	44	45	400	16	1.3	1.2	1.6	3.0
	15-18	54	119	162	65	2,100	48	45	400	14	1.4	1.1	2.0	3.0
	19-22	58	128	162	65	2,100	46	45	400	14	1.4	1.1	2.0	3.0
	23-50	58	128	162	65	2,000	46	45	400	13	1.2	1.0	2.0	3.0
	51+	58	128	162	65	1,800	46	45	400	12	1.1	1.0	2.0	3.0
Pregnant						+300	+30	60	800	+2	+0.3	+0.3	2.5	4.0
Lactating						+500	+20	80	600	+4	+0.5	+0.3	2.5	4.0

[a] The allowances are intended to provide for individual variations among most normal persons as they live in the United States under their usual environmental stresses. Diets should be based on a variety of common foods in order to provide other nutrients for which human requirements have been less well defined.

[b] Kilojoules (kJ) = 4.2 X kcal.

[f] The folacin allowances refer to dietary sources as determined by *Lactobacillus casei* assay. Pure forms of folacin may be effective in doses less than one fourth of the recommended dietary allowance.

[g] Although allowances are expressed as niacin, it is recognized that on the average 1 mg of niacin is derived from each 60 mg of dietary tryptophan.

Eating Right Is Up to You

FOOD AND NUTRITION BOARD, NATIONAL ACADEMY OF SCIENCES-NATIONAL RESEARCH COUNCIL RECOMMENDED DAILY DIETARY ALLOWANCES,[a] Revised 1974 (CONTINUED)

	Age (years)	Weight (kg)	Weight (lbs)	Height (cm)	Height (in)	Energy (kcal)[b]	Protein (g)	Calcium (mg)	Phosphorus (mg)	Iodine (μg)	Iron (mg)	Magnesium (mg)	Zinc (mg)
Infants	0.0-0.5	6	14	60	24	kg × 117	kg × 2.2	360	240	35	10	60	3
	0.5-1.0	9	20	71	28	kg × 108	kg × 2.0	540	400	45	15	70	5
Children	1-3	13	28	86	34	1,300	23	800	800	60	15	150	10
	4-6	20	44	110	44	1,800	30	800	800	80	10	200	10
	7-10	30	66	135	54	2,400	36	800	800	110	10	250	10
Males	11-14	44	97	158	63	2,800	44	1,200	1,200	130	18	350	15
	15-18	61	134	172	69	3,000	54	1,200	1,200	150	18	400	15
	19-22	67	147	172	69	3,000	54	800	800	140	10	350	15
	23-50	70	154	172	69	2,700	56	800	800	130	10	350	15
	51+	70	154	172	69	2,400	56	800	800	110	10	350	15
Females	11-14	44	97	155	62	2,400	44	1,200	1,200	115	18	300	15
	15-18	54	119	162	65	2,100	48	1,200	1,200	115	18	300	15
	19-22	58	128	162	65	2,100	46	800	800	100	18	300	15
	23-50	58	128	162	65	2,000	46	800	800	100	18	300	15
	51+	58	128	162	65	1,800	46	800	800	80	10	300	15
Pregnant						+300	+30	1,200	1,200	125	18+[h]	450	20
Lactating						+500	+20	1,200	1,200	150	18	450	25

[a] The allowances are intended to provide for individual variations among most normal persons as they live in the United States under the usual environmental stresses. Diets should be based on a variety of common foods in order to provide other nutrients for which human requirements have been less well defined.

[b] Kilojoules (kJ) = 4.2 × kcal.

[h] This increased requirement cannot be met by ordinary diets; therefore, the use of supplemental iron is recomended.

(Published with permission.)

Eating Right Is Up to You

THE U.S. RDA FOR ADULTS AND CHILDREN OVER FOUR

Nutrients which *must* be included in Nutrition Information panel		**Nutrients which *may* be included in Nutrition Information panel**	
Nutrient	**U.S. RDA**	**Nutrient**	**U.S. RDA**
Protein	65 g*	Vitamin D	400 IU
Vitamin C	60 mg	Vitamin E	30 IU
Vitamin A	5,000 IU	Vitamin B_6	2 mg
Thiamine**	1.5 mg	Folacin	0.4 mg
Riboflavin	1.7 mg	Vitamin B_{12}	6 μg
Niacin	20 mg	Biotin	0.3 mg
Calcium	1 g	Pantothenic acid	10 mg
Iron	18 mg	Phosphorus	1,000 mg
		Iodine	150 μg
		Zinc	15 mg
		Copper	2 mg

* *The value for protein may vary, depending upon the quality of protein in a specific food.*

** *The Food and Drug Administration uses the spelling "thiamine" rather than the more common spelling "thiamin."*

The Story of Vitamins

It would seem, by vitamins' first given-name category, that they were considered incidentals in food make-up. But, to the contrary, Sir Frederick G. Hopkins, an English biochemist, reported in 1906 that these "accessory factors" were essential substances contained in foods. He found that mice fed purified preparations of recognized essential nutrients couldn't survive. But when mice were given small amounts of milk or certain dried vegetables in addition to the purified diet, they stayed healthy. The substances missing in the purified foods but present in the milk and vegetables were the accessory factors.

The Story of Vitamins

In 1912 Casimir Funk, a Polish scientist working at the Lister Institute in London, coined the word "vitamine" to describe these factors. The word implied that the substances were essential for life (*vita*) and that they belonged to the class of organic compounds known as "amines." The specific factor that Funk was investigating—vitamin B_1 (thiamin)—is an amine, but it was soon learned that not all of these essential factors were amines. Consequently, the terminal "e" was dropped from the spelling of vitamin. The name still reflects the essential life-giving features the substances contain.

Vitamins Identified

Vitamins are organic compounds needed in small amounts in the diet to promote growth and to maintain life. Most vitamins cannot be made in the body, but must be supplied from an outside source through the diet. Exceptions to this include biotin and vitamin K. Both are manufactured by bacteria present in the intestinal tract. The bacteria represent the "outside source," rather than the food we eat. (Vitamin D can be made in the body also, but often not enough is manufactured.)

The words "in small amounts" included in the definition of vitamins serve to distinguish them from the other classes of essential organic compounds. Proteins, fats, and carbohydrates also are organic compounds, but the required amounts are considerably greater than those of vitamins.

Much of the early research leading to the discovery of individual vitamins was carried out with experimental animals. One thing that was discovered was that not all species have the same vitamin requirements. For instance, human beings, monkeys, and guinea pigs need a dietary supply of vitamin C. But most other animal species can manufacture all the vitamin C they need.

Researchers who discovered vitamin A noted that it was present only in the fats and oils of foods; in other words, it

The Story of Vitamins

was soluble in fat. Other investigators found that the B-vitamins were present only in the portion of foods which were soluble in water. So vitamins have been divided into two general groups: the fat-soluble vitamins (vitamins A, D, E, and K) and the water-soluble vitamins (members of the B-complex group and vitamin C).

As vitamins were discovered but before these essential nutrients were chemically identified, they were designated by letters, assigned in alphabetical order. It turned out, however, that the substances first called vitamin A and vitamin B were not single compounds; they were mixtures of compounds. In the case of vitamin B, or as some called it, "water-soluble B," numerical subscripts were added to distinguish individual vitamins as they were discovered, so now we have vitamin B_1, vitamin B_2, vitamin B_6, etc.

Alphabetical designations are still in common use, although names more indicative of a vitamin's chemical nature also are available. But there are missing letters, and some numerical subscripts are not consecutive. The reason is that during the heyday of vitamin research some substances were isolated, thought to have vitamin properties, and given a letter name. When these substances failed to fulfill the criteria for vitamin classification, the name was dropped. Occasionally, too, a new vitamin turned out to be one already discovered and named.

Vitamin Function

As "regulatory nutrients," vitamins direct the flow of chemical reactions involved in the body's use of other nutrients, helping the body to use proteins, fats, and carbohydrates in the proper way to produce energy, promote growth, and maintain good health. Research being done in the area of molecular biology has helped to explain the precise way in which vitamins function. Using sophisticated techniques, scientists in this rapidly developing field can study chemical reactions that take place inside the body cells.

The Story of Vitamins

Many vitamins, especially those of the B-complex group, act as coenzymes. An enzyme is an organic catalyst. It is a biologically active molecule that regulates a specific chemical reaction within the body. All enzymes contain a large protein molecule called an apoenzyme. In addition, many have another, smaller organic molecule attached to the protein which is called a coenzyme. Both the protein and its coenzyme (often a vitamin) are necessary for the enzyme to be active, to carry out its special function.

Much remains to be learned—particularly about the fat-soluble vitamins—about how vitamins function to regulate body chemistry. Research continues.

So Much From So Little

Enzymes control the speed of a chemical reaction, but they are not changed in the process. So vitamins, acting as coenzymes, can be used over and over again by the body. This fact helps to explain why only small amounts of these essential nutrients are needed. Nevertheless, some vitamins are water-soluble and are excreted in the urine, and some are broken down or changed by chemical reactions. So the body needs a regular supply of vitamins to replace those lost or destroyed.

The body recognizes when it has enough of some vitamins. For example, when a water-soluble vitamin is supplied in larger amounts than needed to meet metabolic needs, the excess is rapidly disposed of. The body does not store large amounts of vitamin C or B-vitamins. Since the fat-soluble vitamins do not dissolve in water, they cannot be excreted in the urine; excess amounts are stored in the body. Water-soluble vitamins must be replaced regularly. Fat-soluble ones do not need to be supplied as regularly or continuously if adequate amounts of them are included in the diet in the long run.

Although most vitamins must be supplied by the foods eaten, the body is also capable of manufacturing certain vitamins if it is supplied with proper compounds from other

The Story of Vitamins

sources. For example, plant foods such as fruits and vegetables don't actually contain vitamin A, but many have "vitamin A activity." Some of the orange-yellow compounds called carotenes, which are present in and give the characteristic color to carrots, squash, and cantaloupes, are converted to vitamin A. Carotenes are therefore precursors of vitamin A, or provitamin A.

The body can make a provitamin D and can even synthesize the vitamin. This synthesis takes place when the skin is exposed to sunlight or some other source of ultraviolet light. However, the amount made in the body may be insufficient to meet its needs, and a dietary source must take up the slack. (See the chapter on vitamin D for details.)

Since vitamins function as regulators, they are needed in relatively small amounts. The Table of Recommended Dietary Allowances (see pages 21 to 23) shows that the advised daily intake of thiamin for a man is only 1.4 milligrams (mg), and that for vitamin B_{12} is only 3.0 micrograms (μg). In contrast the RDA for protein for a man is 56 grams (g) per day or about two ounces.

People vary in their needs for vitamins. The RDAs have been set at levels higher than estimated average needs. Thus the requirements of essentially all healthy, normal people are met by the RDAs.

Special Vitamin Needs

During various periods of life and due to various causes, our vitamin needs change. Stress and chronic illness may alter needs for some nutrients; infectious disease can increase the body's requirement for some vitamins but not others. And ailments of the intestinal tract can interfere with the absorption of vitamins causing deficiencies.

In addition, there are people with inherited disorders whose vitamin requirements are quite different from those of healthy individuals. These disorders may hamper the ability of the body to use a vitamin efficiently. For people

The Story of Vitamins

with these conditions, the RDAs have little meaning, and their individual requirements must be evaluated on an individual basis by a physician.

Synthetic versus Natural

Vitamins that are present in foods are natural. Those that are chemically created are referred to as synthetic. Both are sold in supplement form.

Plants are efficient natural vitamin factories. Some of the organic compounds they make to promote their own growth are the very vitamins we need for human health and growth. Also, certain of the bacteria which belong to the plant kingdom are helpful in making and supplying vitamins for people. Plant products even reach us through the meat and dairy foods we eat. Through these foods, we obtain the vitamins from the plants the animals have eaten.

A vitamin is not always a single compound, however. The vitamin E value of a food, for instance, is supplied by several different compounds, each of which has vitamin E activity, and vitamin B_6 activity is contributed by at least three different substances. The compounds which make up vitamin E or vitamin B_6 have similar chemical structures. Presumably, they function in much the same way, or they may be converted to a single active compound in the body. (Synthetic vitamins are often patterned after the form of the vitamin with the highest biological activity or the one most easily absorbed by the intestine.)

Vitamins used to enrich or fortify foods and those present in many supplements are synthetic. They are made from simpler compounds or starting materials by controlled chemical reactions. In a sense they are products of the laboratory as opposed to being products of nature.

For some, the word "synthetic" suggests inferiority. Synthetic vitamins are often down-graded and considered of less value than natural. Some people even argue that synthetic vitamins are potentially dangerous since coal tar products are sometimes used as starting materials for their

The Story of Vitamins

manufacture. Many coal tar products are poisonous and some can cause cancer, but the final product, the synthetic vitamin, is highly purified.

It has been suggested also that natural vitamin supplements may contain other unidentified compounds which may be useful or even essential to human health. The possibility does exist that more vitamins may yet be discovered, but these unidentified vitamins must be required in miniscule amounts because no evidence of deficiency diseases which respond to specific foods or natural vitamin supplements has been found.

Essentially, a vitamin is a vitamin, regardless of its source. With respect to its chemical structure, a vitamin made by a growing plant is identical to one made by a drug company, and the body can't tell the difference.

Early Research

Disease conditions caused by vitamin deficiencies were known long before the first vitamin was discovered. The ability of some foods to prevent or cure certain of these diseases has also been known for centuries.

In 400 B.C. Hippocrates described symptoms of a disease which today is known as scurvy, a vitamin C deficiency. The debilitating effects and the many deaths caused by scurvy were recorded in the log books of 15th- and 16th-century explorers. In 1747, Dr. James Lind, a physician in the British navy, showed that oranges and lemons could cure the disease. Giving a variety of foods to sick sailors, he found that only those men who received the citrus fruits recovered quickly. However, it wasn't until 50 years later that the British navy included lime juice in her ships' stores for use by the crew to prevent scurvy.

Lind's investigation was one of the first nutrition experiments to use human subjects. The search for the cause of and cure for certain diseases in people and in experimental animals contributed to the eventual discovery and identification of vitamins.

The Story of Vitamins

Progress was slow. People had difficulty accepting the concept that diseases could be caused by the lack of something in the foods they ate. The scientific community resisted the concept even more following Louis Pasteur's discovery of bacteria. Investigators who were studying the deficiency diseases often had to prove, first, that the maladies were not caused by infectious bacteria, then, second, that the diseases were caused by a deficiency of an essential nutrient.

Subclinical Deficiency

When the amount of a nutrient in the diet or the total "body pool" of a nutrient is only marginally adequate, the condition is called a "subclinical deficiency." Biochemical and metabolic changes begin to take place, and an individual with this condition is considered to be "at risk." Outward signs of deficiency are not apparent, but symptoms can develop rapidly if the nutrient intake suddenly drops or if the person's nutrient requirement suddenly increases due to physiological stress.

Identification of subclinical vitamin deficiency can only be confirmed by laboratory tests. Such tests include measurement of the amount of the vitamin in the blood and the amount excreted in the urine. In some instances metabolic derivatives of a vitamin are measured. In other cases certain compounds tend to accumulate when the vitamin necessary for their further metabolism is in low supply. The amount of these compounds in the blood or urine is indicative of the vitamin status of the individual. It is also possible to measure the activity of certain enzymes which require vitamins as coenzymes. For example, the enzyme known as transketolase (present in red blood cells) has a below-normal degree of activity when the supply of thiamin, its coenzyme, is limited.

The degree of risk of any subclinical deficiency can vary widely from an almost total exhaustion of a specific vitamin supply to only a slight below-normal balance. For this

The Story of Vitamins

reason it is often difficult to detect any effect on a person's health due to a subclinical vitamin deficiency. When such a lack is identified, however, it suggests that the person's diet needs improving and, in some instances, calls for the use of supplementary vitamins.

Vitamin Toxicity

A vitamin toxicity can be as serious as a deficiency. Vitamins A and D can accumulate in the body as a result of taking large doses over a long period of time. The toxicity produced by excesses of these two vitamins is well documented. (See the chapters devoted to these vitamins for details.)

Toxicity due to long-term use of high doses of the other eleven vitamins has not been clearly established. There is evidence, however, that high intakes of some may have undesirable effects at least for some individuals. Also, a vitamin imbalance could occur. Taking excessive amounts of one vitamin could conceivably cause a deficiency of another even though the second vitamin is being consumed in amounts which would be adequate ordinarily. For example, animal studies have shown that high doses of vitamin E may adversely affect the status of vitamin K.

Research into vitamin toxicity continues. At present there are many unanswered questions about the use of megadoses of vitamins. The term "megadose" refers to an amount at least ten times the RDA.

Therapeutic Use and Vitamins as Drugs

Vitamin deficiencies require vitamin therapy. As a result of poor eating habits, inadequate diets, pathological conditions involving poor absorption or utilization of vitamins, or an increase in a vitamin requirement, a person may become vitamin deficient and require treatment. A deficiency caused by poor eating habits obviously is best treated by correcting the diet to take in more of the foods

The Story of Vitamins

which provide the vitamin that is in low supply. Vitamin deficiencies that are the result of a disease condition need careful evaluation by a physician who will treat the disease and the deficiency. Whatever the cause, vitamin supplements that provide two to five times the RDAs are usually indicated for treatment of a deficiency.

Currently there is widespread promotion of "megavitamin therapy," or "orthomolecular therapy" (see the chapter on megavitamin therapy). Promotion is based on the premise that large doses of vitamins are useful for the prevention, treatment, or cure of many diseases. For example, vitamin C is promoted for the prevention and treatment of the common cold and vitamin E for heart disease. Most of these claims have not been substantiated by carefully controlled experimental studies, however.

Large doses of some vitamins do have some biological or metabolic effects. For example, nicotinic acid (a form of niacin) in large amounts reduces the level of cholesterol in the blood. But any possible drug-like action of a vitamin is unrelated to its nutritional function. It is not acting as a nutrient because the amount given is much more than is needed to meet nutritional requirements. It is being used as a drug.

There is no nutritionally sound basis for using megadoses of vitamins as "insurance" against possible dietary shortages. Supplements with vitamins in amounts much greater than the RDA should not be used without medical supervision. Self-treatment of real or suspected diseases with massive doses of vitamins is potentially hazardous. Some vitamins are known to be toxic when consumed in large amounts. Self-diagnosis and self-treatment can only delay appropriate medical attention.

Vitamin Supplements

There are three classifications for the great variety of vitamin preparations available today: prescription drugs, nonprescription or over-the-counter (OTC) drugs, and

The Story of Vitamins

dietary supplements. Prescription drugs can be purchased only with a physician's prescription. They are controlled by the Food and Drug Administration (FDA) under rules and regulations applicable to all drugs. The second class, OTC vitamin drug products, can be purchased without prescription, but they, too, are subject to the regulatory authority of the FDA. According to law, products are considered drugs if they are intended for use "in the diagnosis, cure, mitigation, treatment, or prevention of disease."

Most vitamin products available today fall into the third class, "dietary supplements." When these are advertised and labeled without claims for intended use against disease they are not subject to regulation by the FDA. A 1976 act of Congress stripped the FDA of most of its authority to control the composition and potency of dietary supplements.

As part of its program for reviewing all nonprescription drugs, the FDA in 1973 appointed an independent advisory panel to review the safety, effectiveness, and labeling of OTC vitamin and mineral drug products. One aspect of FDA control of drugs is the requirement that they be proved safe and effective for their intended use. The final report of the advisory panel was published on March 16, 1979 in the *Federal Register,* together with FDA proposals for regulation of OTC vitamin-mineral drug preparations. The panel concluded that representation of any such products for use in the prevention or treatment of a vitamin or mineral deficiency is a claim for therapeutic use, and requires that the products be considered drugs. As it stands, some of the current advertising for dietary supplements comes close to being this type of a representation.

The recommendations of the panel, upon which the rules proposed by the FDA are based, came only after several years of review and evaluation. The panel's conclusions have served as useful guidelines to the editors of CONSUMER GUIDE® magazine in making their recommendations relative to use of vitamin supplements. While the panel addressed itself only to OTC drug

The Story of Vitamins

products, it is our judgment that no additional benefits for prevention or treatment of vitamin deficiencies can be expected from use of dietary supplements containing vitamins at levels or potencies higher than those recommended for OTC drug products. Further, we agree with the panel that the inclusion of nonvitamin substances in vitamin supplements serves no useful purpose.

Nonvitamins

Compounds classified as vitamins must meet certain criteria. First, a deficiency of the substance must eventually produce characteristic deficiency symptoms. Second, the deficiency symptoms produced should be reversed or cured when the compound is supplied. But there are exceptions to the second criterion. For example, long-term deficiency of vitamin A causes irreversible damage to the eye, eventually leading to blindness. In general, however, the 13 compounds now classified as vitamins essential for humans meet these criteria.

During early vitamin-research studies, a number of compounds were isolated from foods and thought to have vitamin properties. Further investigation revealed that some of these substances were vitamins for certain animals, but not for humans.

Choline, inositol, and p-aminobenzoic acid (PABA) were once considered vitamins for man. These substances can be synthesized by the human body, however, and a lack of them in the diet does not cause deficiency symptoms. In seriously ill persons, the mechanisms for making these compounds may not function properly, and a supplemental supply may be helpful.

These three compounds are included in many multivitamin supplements, especially those sold in health food stores. They are also available as individual supplements in amounts varying over a wide range.

Adelle Davis made many claims for PABA. In *Let's Eat Right To Keep Fit* she stated that PABA has anti-graying

The Story of Vitamins

properties.[1] Some animals require a dietary source of PABA, and when they are deprived of it dark hair turns gray. However, any claim that PABA can reverse graying in humans is not supported by any scientific evidence. Davis also recommended PABA supplements for treating eczema and parasitic diseases such as Rocky Mountain spotted fever and typhus as well as for protection against sunburn.

To correct baldness, Davis recommended that a person drink a quart of milk to which was added a teaspoon of pure inositol. She also recommended choline for the treatment of nephritis and kidney disease. (A brochure from the Windmill Natural Vitamin Company further claims that choline and inositol retard hardening of the arteries.) Sales of these nonvitamins go on, but there is no evidence to support any of these claims.

Other nonvitamins often incorporated into multivitamin supplements include rutin, lipoic acid, bioflavonoids, and hesperidin. The term "complete vitamin C complex" may be used to describe a combination of the vitamin and bioflavonoids which come from the peels of citrus fruits. In *Linda Clark's Handbook of Natural Remedies for Common Ailments,* it is suggested that people using supplements of the entire complex could develop immunity to allergies, notably hay fever and poison oak or ivy.[2] There are no data to support this premise.

Claims have been made recently for the controversial anticancer substance, laetrile, which is referred to as vitamin B_{17}. Apparently, proponents of the substance call it a vitamin to avoid its classification and regulation as a drug. There is no evidence to warrant giving vitamin status to laetrile.

One of the latest additions to the list of nonvitamins is pangamic acid, erroneously labeled vitamin B_{15}. Dr. Alan Cott, a New York psychiatrist, reports that autistic children become gregarious and sociable after taking doses of vitamin B_{15}. Cott also claims dramatic success with megavitamin therapy in treating children with learning

The Story of Vitamins

disabilities. No data have been set forth to support these claims, however.

The current widespread promotion of nonvitamin supplements raises false hopes for treatment or cure of serious diseases. The premise that people who consume ordinary diets may be deficient in nonvitamin substances is contradicted by scientific evidence which shows that these substances are not essential to a person's well-being. To pay for what you don't need is clearly a waste of money.

Only the 13 compounds discussed in the following chapters are considered essential vitamins for human health, although future research may raise other substances to vitamin status. Until then, the guidelines are clear, and the claims remain unfounded.

Thiamin (Vitamin B₁)

The discovery of thiamin (vitamin B_1) in the 1930s marked the end of the story of a disease, a disease born of technology.

Beriberi, a debilitating and often fatal ailment, did not become a serious health problem among the rice-eating peoples of the Orient until the end of the 19th century. At that time, mills began to polish rice to remove the outer, brown layers of the grain and produce smooth white kernels. When the rice was stripped of its bran, it lost much of the thiamin it contained. People who ate the polished rice were deprived of this vitamin, and the incidence of beriberi rose to an epidemic level. A similar situation arose

Thiamin (Vitamin B$_1$)

in countries where wheat was a staple food and refined white flour began to replace whole-wheat flour.

Before mills made refined grains available to many people, beriberi was uncommon. With the rise of commercial milling of rice and other cereals came a swift increase in prevalence of the disease. The increased prevalence spurred efforts to find the cause of and cure for beriberi. Still, the search took almost 50 years. It did not end until the vitamin thiamin was discovered.

History

K. Takaki, a medical officer in the Japanese navy, was the first to suspect that diet had a bearing on beriberi. In the 1880s, Takaki sought the root of this disease, which afflicted large numbers of Japanese sailors on long voyages. The disease was so rampant that on one nine-month voyage, 169 of the 276 crew members aboard one ship developed beriberi, and 25 of them died. To test his belief that diet was at fault, Takaki added meat and milk to the rice diet provided to sailors. He found that during a similar voyage only a few men—just those who had refused to eat the meat and milk—came down with the malady.

Further evidence of the relationship between diet and beriberi came from Java, where the Dutch physician Christiaan Eijkman found that chickens fed polished rice exhibited symptoms similar to those of beriberi. When he fed the chickens unpolished rice, the symptoms disappeared. Eijkman extended his experiments to humans and confirmed that beriberi could be prevented or cured if unpolished rice were substituted for polished grain.

The explanation for these findings was not put forward until 1901, when Gerrit Grijns, a nutrition researcher also working in Java, suggested that unpolished rice contained an unknown substance that prevented beriberi. In 1910 chemist Robert Williams began a similar search. While working in the Philippines, he was asked by a member of

Thiamin (Vitamin B$_1$)

the U.S. Army Medical Corps to analyze a brown liquid that had been extracted from rice polishings. Williams painstakingly tested the substances from the liquid for their effect on polyneuritis, a disease among chickens which is similar to beriberi. It was 1934 before Williams isolated the substance that acted against beriberi. It was the vitamin thiamin.[1]

Food Sources of Thiamin

As Williams found in his search for the vitamin, thiamin is present in tiny amounts in most foods. Some foods are better sources of thiamin than others. About 70 percent of the thiamin in the American diet comes equally from the cereal and meat groups. Enriched and whole-grain cereal products are good sources of the vitamin, and pork is an especially rich source. (See the first table at the end of this chapter for the thiamin content of some common foods.)

Thiamin is not a stable compound. It can be destroyed by exposure to high temperatures and, because it is water-soluble, can be leached from foods in their cooking water. So to prevent loss of the vitamin, foods should be prepared in the least amount of water at the lowest possible temperature for the shortest period of time.

Dietary Requirements for Thiamin

The Recommended Dietary Allowance (RDA) for thiamin is related to calorie intake and allows 0.50 mg of thiamin for every 1,000 calories. Human beings, depending on whether they live sedentary or physically active lives, have different calorie needs and different needs for thiamin. The RDA for mildly active men is 1.4 mg. Mildly active women have an RDA of 1.0 mg. The Food and Nutrition Board suggests that, even when the calorie intake is under 2,000, the thiamin intake should not fall below 1.0 mg.[2]

Most people should have no trouble meeting the RDA for thiamin in their diets. To get an idea of how the thiamin

Thiamin (Vitamin B$_1$)

content in two typical diets compares with the RDA, and for a list of good food sources and the percent of the U.S. RDA for thiamin provided by those foods, see the second and third tables at the end of this chapter. Because calorie needs are greater during the last three months of pregnancy and while a woman is nursing, the Food and Nutrition Board recommends that women increase their daily intake of thiamin by 0.30 mg during these times.

Function of Thiamin

Like other B-complex vitamins, thiamin acts as a biologic catalyst, or coenzyme. As a coenzyme, thiamin participates in the long chain of reactions that provide energy for the body to function and heat for the body to maintain a constant temperature. Thiamin also is involved in the synthesis of fats and in protein metabolism.

Deficiency of Thiamin

In an East Indian dialect, beriberi means weakness; and weakness is a chief symptom of one form of the disease: the so-called dry type of beriberi. Dry beriberi is characterized by numbness, muscle weakness, loss of appetite, and disorders of the nervous system which restrict a person's coordination and cause difficulty in walking. In contrast, wet beriberi is characterized by an accumulation of water in the body, especially in the legs. This severe form of the disease interferes with the normal function of the heart and the circulatory system and may eventually cause heart failure.

   Severe thiamin deficiency seldom occurs today in the Western world. Alcoholics who eat little or no food for extended periods of time may develop symptoms of beriberi, and children who are in a state of starvation may have the disease. Otherwise, the amount of thiamin in an ordinary mixed diet is sufficient to prevent severe deficiency.

Thiamin (Vitamin B$_1$)

The amount of thiamin in the diet might not be sufficient to prevent what is termed a subclinical deficiency, however. A subclinical deficiency occurs when the amount of a particular nutrient in the diet or in the body is barely adequate. Such a deficiency does not produce symptoms, but it can be confirmed by certain laboratory tests. For example, it may show up in tests that measure the concentration of thiamin in the blood, determine the amount of thiamin or its metabolic products in the urine, or analyze the compounds that depend on thiamin for their metabolism. The number of people with a subclinical thiamin deficiency in the United States is unknown. What is known is that intakes of the vitamin ranging from 0.35 mg to 0.45 mg for every 1,000 calories are adequate for good health. So if you meet the RDA of 0.50 mg for every 1,000 calories, you'll have a 40 percent margin of safety against subclinical deficiency.

On the other side of the world, beriberi is a common cause of death in infants. Frequently, women in the Orient subsist on thiamin-deficient diets. So when they are nursing they cannot provide enough of the vitamin for their infants, and the infants develop beriberi in the first few months of life. The beriberi that occurs in Eastern countries nowadays is not due to thiamin deficiency alone. Diets based on a single staple such as rice usually are low or deficient in other nutrients as well, and some of the symptoms of beriberi are associated with this lack.

Therapeutic Uses of Thiamin

Doses of two to five times the RDA are effective in treating thiamin deficiency. Only a physician can determine if a true thiamin deficiency exists. One or two milligrams of supplemental thiamin are enough to prevent deficiency.

Hazards and Toxicity of Thiamin

Studies with animals showed that massive doses of

Thiamin (Vitamin B$_1$)

thiamin were lethal when injected intravenously. However, studies conducted on humans indicated that thiamin in doses of up to 200 times the RDA were not toxic when injected intravenously or intramuscularly. Other studies showed that large doses of thiamin taken by mouth caused no toxicity or adverse effects in humans.

Claims and Controversy

Thiamin has been touted for its "energy-giving" properties and for its ability to get rid of that "tired, run-down feeling." However, thiamin cannot provide instant energy. Thiamin plays a part in the chain of reactions that supplies the body with energy; but by itself it cannot provide energy, and it has no effect on fatigue in the absence of deficiency. Thiamin deficiency causes loss of appetite, but that does not mean extra amounts of the vitamin will stimulate the appetite.

Among the other conditions for which beneficial claims have been made are: dermatitis, multiple sclerosis, neuritis, and mental disorders. The Advisory Panel on Vitamin and Mineral Drug Products for Over-the-Counter Human Use[3] concluded that thiamin supplements are of no benefit in the treatment of any of these symptoms or diseases in which there is no evidence of a thiamin deficiency.

CONSUMER GUIDE® magazine Opinion

By following the RDA, you should be able to get enough thiamin to meet your body's needs.

Thiamin Summary

Type of vitamin: Water-soluble
Where stored in the body: The body does not store excess amounts of thiamin.
History: Isolated in 1926; chemical structure determined in 1934

Thiamin (Vitamin B_1)

Food sources: Cereals (whole-grain and enriched products) and meats; especially pork

Recommended Dietary Allowance: 1.4 mg for men; 1.0 mg for women, based on 0.50 mg per 1,000 calories

Function: Thiamin helps the body produce energy and heat, and assists in the metabolism of carbohydrates, fats, and proteins.

Deficiency: Results in beriberi

Therapeutic uses: Physicians prescribe supplements to treat thiamin deficiency.

Hazards and toxicity: No toxicity or undesirable side effect has followed the use of large doses of thiamin by humans.

Claims and controversy: Thiamin has been touted for its "energy-producing" properties and its ability to end that "tired, run-down feeling." But thiamin by itself cannot supply energy. Thiamin cannot stimulate the appetite, even though thiamin deficiency does cause loss of appetite. Thiamin supplements are ineffective against dermatitis, multiple sclerosis, neuritis or mental disorders.

CONSUMER GUIDE® magazine opinion: Eat a variety of foods and follow the RDA.

Thiamin (Vitamin B_1)

THIAMIN CONTENT OF COMMON FOODS

Food	Quantity	Milligrams of Thiamin
Milk Group		
Milk, whole or skim	1 cup	0.09
Yogurt	1 cup	0.08
Cottage cheese	1 cup	0.05
Ice cream	1 cup	0.05
Meat Group		
Pork roast	3 ounces	0.78
Pork chop, cooked	1	0.63
Ham	3 ounces	0.40
Dry beans, peas; cooked	1 cup	0.25
Peanuts	½ cup	0.23
Beef liver	3 ounces	0.22
Bologna	2 slices	0.10
Frankfurter	1	0.08
Ground beef	3 ounces	0.07
Roast beef	3 ounces	0.05
Chicken	3 ounces	0.04
Fish	3 ounces	0.03 to 0.06
Fruit and Vegetable Group		
Peas, cooked	½ cup	0.22
Orange	1 medium	0.13
Asparagus	½ cup	0.11
Orange juice	4 ounces	0.11
Potatoes		
Baked	1 medium	0.10
French fries	10 pieces	0.07
Chips	10 pieces	0.04
Iceberg lettuce	¼ head	0.08
Banana	1 medium	0.06
Cabbage, raw	1 cup	0.05
Green or snap beans	½ cup	0.05
Apple	1 medium	0.04
Carrot, raw	1 medium	0.04

Thiamin (Vitamin B$_1$)

THIAMIN CONTENT OF COMMON FOODS

Food	Quantity	Milligrams of Thiamin
Cereal Group		
Ready-to-eat breakfast cereals (enriched)		
Total, Product 19	1 ounce each	1.50
King Vitaman	1 ounce	0.90
Wheaties, corn flakes, Bran Flakes	1 ounce each	0.37
Rice; enriched, cooked	1 cup	0.23
Macaroni, noodles, spaghetti; cooked, enriched	1 cup	0.20
Bread, white enriched	1 slice	0.10
Bread, whole-wheat	1 slice	0.06

Compiled from: product labels and U.S.D.A. *Home and Garden Bulletin No. 72,* Washington, D.C., revised April, 1977.

Thiamin (Vitamin B$_1$)

THIAMIN CONTENT IN TWO DAILY DIETS

Typical Day's Diet for Woman (1,700 Calories)	Milligrams of Thiamin
Breakfast	
4 ounces orange juice	0.11
1 ounce enriched corn flakes	0.37
1 slice enriched white toast	0.10
1 pat butter	none
1 cup 2-percent milk	0.08
Black coffee	none
Lunch	
Sandwich: 2 slices whole-wheat bread, 1 slice American cheese, 2 ounces boiled ham	0.37
1 cup skim milk	0.09
½ cup cole slaw	0.04
Dinner	
½ chicken breast, fried	0.04
1 medium baked potato	0.10
1 cup tossed green salad	0.05
½ cup peas, cooked	0.22
1 enriched dinner roll	0.10
2 pats butter	none
½ cup ice cream	0.03
Black coffee	none
Total	**1.70**
RDA	**1.00**

Compiled from: U.S.D.A. *Home and Garden Bulletin No. 72,* Washington, D.C., revised April, 1977.

Thiamin (Vitamin B$_1$)

THIAMIN CONTENT IN TWO DAILY DIETS

Typical Day's Diet for Teenage Boy (3,000 Calories)	Milligrams of Thiamin
Breakfast	
½ medium pink grapefruit	0.05
2 scrambled eggs	0.10
2 slices enriched white toast	0.20
1 pat butter	none
1 cup whole milk	0.09
Lunch	
1 cheeseburger	0.22
2 cups whole milk	0.18
10 large French-fried potatoes	0.07
1 medium banana	0.06
Dinner	
4 ounces round steak	0.09
1 cup green beans	0.10
1 cup mashed potatoes	0.16
Lettuce and tomato salad	0.05
2 slices enriched white bread	0.20
1 pat butter	none
1 cup whole milk	0.09
4 chocolate chip cookies	0.04
Snacks	
Cola drink	none
½ cup ice cream	0.03
¼ of 14-inch cheese pizza	0.08
Total	**1.81**
RDA	**1.50**

Compiled from: U.S.D.A. *Home and Garden Bulletin No. 72,* Washington, D.C., revised April, 1977.

Thiamin (Vitamin B$_1$)

GOOD SOURCES OF THIAMIN

This table lists a variety of foods that are good sources of thiamin. Thiamin is present in tiny amounts in most foods. About 70 percent of the thiamin in the American diet comes equally from the cereal and meat groups. Enriched and whole-grain cereal products are good sources and pork is an especially rich source of the vitamin. The U.S. RDA for adults and children over four for thiamin is 1.5 mg.

Food	Quantity	Percent of U.S. RDA
Product 19 breakfast cereal	1 ounce	100.00
Total breakfast cereal	1 ounce	100.00
Pistachio nuts	1 cup	62.67
Pecan halves	1 cup	62.00
Pork roast	3 ounces	52.00
Oatmeal, ready-to-serve	¾ cup	50.73
Filberts or hazelnuts	1 cup	42.67
Pork chop, cooked	1 chop (3½ ounces)	42.00
Cashews, roasted	1 cup	40.00
Macadamia nuts	1 cup	32.00
Peas; green, cooked	1 cup	29.33
Spareribs, braised	3½ ounces	28.67
Ham, roasted	3 ounces	26.67
Wheaties breakfast cereal	1 ounce	24.67
Dry beans, peas; cooked	1 cup	16.67
Peanuts	½ cup	15.33
Rice; enriched, cooked	1 cup	15.33
Beef liver	3 ounces	14.67
Orange juice	1 cup	14.67
Bread, white enriched	2 slices	13.33
Macaroni, noodles, spaghetti; cooked, enriched	1 cup	13.33
Orange	1 medium	8.67
Bread, whole-wheat	2 slices	8.00
Potato, baked	1 medium	6.67

Thiamin (Vitamin B$_1$)

GOOD SOURCES OF THIAMIN

Food	Quantity	Percent of U.S. RDA
Milk, whole or skim	1 cup	6.00
Pumpernickel bread	2 slices	5.78
Rye bread	2 slices	5.78
Frankfurter	1	5.33
Yogurt	1 cup	5.33
Ground beef	3 ounces	4.67
Cottage cheese	1 cup	3.33
Chicken	3 ounces	2.67
Fish	3 ounces	2.00-4.00

Compiled from: CONSUMER GUIDE® magazine Nutrition Data Bank.

Riboflavin (Vitamin B₂)

Riboflavin's story is a colorful one—it's yellow in fact. In the 1920s and 1930s nutritionists were searching for a growth-promoting factor in food, and they kept finding yellow substances. Meanwhile, biochemists were trying to solve some of the mysteries of metabolism, and they kept running into a yellow enzyme. The yellow substances in foods and part of the enzyme were both riboflavin.

History

Most nutritionists in the 1920s believed that there were only two unidentified essential nutrients, a fat-soluble "A"

Riboflavin (Vitamin B$_2$)

and a water-soluble "B." Soon, however, they found that there was a second water-soluble B compound. So the researchers set to the task of identifying that other B compound.

They gradually separated growth-producing substances from liver, eggs, milk, and grass and found that all the substances were yellow. In 1933 L.E. Booher reported that she had obtained a yellow, growth-promoting substance from milk whey. She observed that the darker the color of the substance, the greater its potency. Booher's observation was a clue that led nutritionists to the discovery that all the yellow growth-producing substances they had found in foods were one and the same: riboflavin.

While nutritionists were zeroing in on the yellow substance in food, biochemists were studying a yellow enzyme that was essential for the body to produce energy. The biochemists could separate the enzyme into two parts: a colorless protein and a yellow organic compound. The yellow compound was riboflavin. The convergence of the two lines of research provided an explanation for the growth-promoting properties of riboflavin and furnished information about its biochemical mechanism. This was the first indication that many of the B vitamins function as coenzymes.

Food Sources of Riboflavin

Milk is the best source of riboflavin in the American diet. A glass of milk provides one-fourth the Recommended Dietary Allowance (RDA) of the vitamin for a man and a third of the RDA for a woman. Other dairy products—cheese, yogurt, and ice cream—are also good sources of the vitamin. Meats, especially organ meats such as liver and kidney, are particularly rich in riboflavin, as are green, leafy vegetables.

Cereals generally are the poorest sources, but they still contribute some riboflavin. A few highly enriched breakfast cereals, however, contain 100 percent of the U.S. RDA for

Riboflavin (Vitamin B$_2$)

adults in a single serving. (See the first two tables at the end of this chapter for the riboflavin content of some common foods and for a list of good food sources of riboflavin and the percent of the U.S. RDA they provide.

The riboflavin present in food can be destroyed by light. To guard against loss of the vitamin, food should be covered, especially during cooking. And milk, the best source of the vitamin, should be kept out of direct sunlight.

Dietary Requirements for Riboflavin

The RDA for riboflavin allows 0.60 mg for every 1,000 calories consumed. This figure translates into a daily allowance for riboflavin of 1.6 mg for men and 1.2 mg for women. (An additional 0.3 mg per day is recommended for pregnant women and 0.5 mg per day for nursing mothers.) The last table at the end of this chapter shows the riboflavin content in two typical daily diets.

Function of Riboflavin

Riboflavin does not act alone in the body; it works in concert with its B-complex kin. Yet riboflavin has specific duties to perform. These duties involve the formation of two complex compounds.

In the body, riboflavin is changed to form compounds known to biochemists as flavinmononucleotide and flavin adenine dinucleotide. These compounds attach to proteins and form enzymes. The enzymes help to metabolize carbohydrates, proteins, and fats to generate energy.

Deficiency of Riboflavin

A dietary lack of the vitamin (ariboflavinosis) stunts the growth of young animals. This is not, however, a specific effect of riboflavin deficiency. Growth failure is also associated with other vitamin deficiencies. Symptoms more specific to ariboflavinosis include angular stomatitis

Riboflavin (Vitamin B$_2$)

(cracks or fissures at the corners of the mouth), cheilosis (inflammation and soreness of the lips), and glossitis (smooth, reddish-purple tongue). Such symptoms have been seen in people whose diets were very low in riboflavin and in experiments with human volunteers maintained on riboflavin-deficient diets.[1,2] Similar symptoms may indicate deficiencies of other vitamins and some trace minerals. In these cases a full nutritional study should be considered.

A deficiency of riboflavin does not have specific symptoms because riboflavin does not act alone in the body. Because the B vitamins work together in a chain of reactions, when one link is weak due to a deficiency of one vitamin it affects the entire chain. Experiments showed that symptoms appeared when diets provided only 0.25 mg of riboflavin for every 1,000 calories. Other studies showed that only one individual in a group of 48 men and women exhibited symptoms of deficiency when the daily intake of the vitamin was 0.35 mg for every 1,000 calories. However, when the intake is that low the body has no riboflavin to spare. Only when the diet provides 0.50 mg or more per 1,000 calories does the body have more of this vitamin than it can use. The RDA allows an extra margin of safety.

Therapeutic Uses of Riboflavin

Physicians prescribe riboflavin doses of as much as two to five times the RDA to treat deficiency. Therapeutic doses of riboflavin have not been shown to be beneficial in the treatment of any other conditions. Multivitamin supplements containing riboflavin are often prescribed for pregnant women to prevent deficiency.

Hazards and Toxicity of Riboflavin

Large doses of riboflavin have not caused toxicity or adverse reactions. Doses as high as 10 grams of the

Riboflavin (Vitamin B$_2$)

vitamin per kilogram of body weight (10 g for every 2.2 pounds) produced no harmful effects in animals. For a 155-pound man, such a dose would be almost 600,000 times the RDA.

Claims and Controversy

Riboflavin has few claims attached to its name. For the most part, the claims have been based on the findings from animal studies.

In animals, prolonged and severe riboflavin deficiency causes extensive eye damage. The suggestion that most cataracts in humans may be caused by riboflavin deficiency seems to stem from this finding. But the probability of such a prolonged deficiency happening to a person is remote, and as yet there are no data to support the connection between riboflavin deficiency and severe eye damage in people. Nor is there evidence that extra riboflavin is effective in treating eye problems.

In *Let's Eat Right to Keep Fit* Adelle Davis said: "It has been my experience that symptoms of [riboflavin] deficiency are to be found in almost every person who drinks less than one quart of milk a day."[3] Although milk is an excellent source of the vitamin, people can easily meet the RDA for riboflavin without drinking milk by the quart. Just one glass supplies one-fourth the RDA for men and one-third the RDA for women.

(Large amounts of riboflavin are included together with other vitamins in a variety of megavitamin programs promoted for prevention, treatment, and cure of various diseases. See the chapter on megavitamin therapy for details.)

CONSUMER GUIDE® magazine Opinion

Most Americans get sufficient riboflavin in their diets to prevent an out-and-out deficiency. CONSUMER GUIDE® magazine recommends that you plan diets to include a

Riboflavin (Vitamin B$_2$)

variety of foods of different classes—especially milk and milk products—to meet your need for riboflavin.

Riboflavin Summary

Type of vitamin: Water-soluble
Where stored in the body: The body does not store excess amounts of riboflavin.
History: Discovered in 1933
Food sources: The best food sources of riboflavin are milk and dairy products, meats, and green, leafy vegetables.
Recommended Dietary Allowance: 1.6 mg for men; 1.2 mg for women, based on 0.60 mg per 1,000 calories
Function: Riboflavin acts as a coenzyme and is essential for energy production.
Deficiency: Linked with other B-vitamin deficiencies; medical examination required.
Therapeutic uses: Prevention and treatment of riboflavin deficiency (ariboflavinosis)
Hazards and toxicity: No toxic or adverse reactions have been reported following large doses of riboflavin.
Claims and controversy: Riboflavin deficiency has caused severe eye damage in experimental animals. This eye damage in animals has followed prolonged deficiency that is unlikely in man. There are no data to support the connection between riboflavin deficiency and serious eye problems in humans.

Although Adelle Davis asserted that each individual should drink a quart of milk a day to avoid riboflavin deficiency, adequate amounts of the vitamin can be obtained from other foods.
CONSUMER GUIDE® magazine opinion: To assure adequate amounts of the vitamin, we advise you to remain aware of the RDA for this vitamin and to include milk and milk products in your daily diets.

Riboflavin (Vitamin B_2)

RIBOFLAVIN CONTENT OF COMMON FOODS

Food	Quantity	Milligrams of Riboflavin
Milk Group		
Milk shake, thick (made from mix)	10 ounces	0.65
Milk, whole or skim	1 cup	0.38
Cottage cheese	1 cup	0.34
Ice cream, ice milk	1 cup	0.33
Yogurt (various types and flavors)	1 cup	0.32-0.53
Cheese, natural and processed	1 ounce	0.11
Meat Group		
Beef liver	3 ounces	3.56
Ground beef	1 hamburger	0.20
Pork chop, cooked	1	0.18
Chicken	3 ounces	0.15
Egg	1 whole	0.15
Ham	3 ounces	0.15
Roast beef	3 ounces	0.15
Peas and beans; dried, cooked	1 cup	0.13
Bologna	2 slices	0.12
Frankfurter	1	0.11
Peanuts	½ cup	0.10
Tuna	3 ounces	0.10
Cereal Group		
Ready-to-eat breakfast cereals (enriched)		
Total, Product 19	1 ounce each	1.70
King Vitaman	1 ounce	1.02
Wheaties, Grape Nuts Flakes, corn flakes	1 ounce each	0.42

Riboflavin (Vitamin B_2)

RIBOFLAVIN CONTENT OF COMMON FOODS

Food	Quantity	Milligrams of Riboflavin
Macaroni, noodles, spaghetti; enriched, cooked	1 cup	0.12
Bread, white enriched	1 slice	0.06
Oatmeal, cooked	1 cup	0.05
Bread, whole-wheat	1 slice	0.03
Rice, cooked	1 cup	0.02
Fruit and Vegetable Group		
Broccoli, cooked	½ cup	0.15
Spinach, cooked	½ cup	0.13
Squash, winter; baked, mashed	½ cup	0.13
Asparagus, cooked	½ cup	0.11
Banana	1 medium	0.07
Potato, baked	1 medium	0.07
Apple	1 medium	0.06
Green or snap beans	½ cup	0.05
Orange	1 medium	0.05
Strawberries, raw	½ cup	0.05
Carrot, raw	1 medium	0.02

Compiled from: product labels and U.S.D.A. *Home and Garden Bulletin No. 72,* Washington, D.C., revised April, 1977.

Riboflavin (Vitamin B$_2$)

GOOD SOURCES OF RIBOFLAVIN

This table lists a variety of foods that are good sources of riboflavin. Milk is the best source of riboflavin in the American diet. Other dairy products are also good sources of the vitamin, as are meats and green, leafy vegetables. Cereals generally are the poorest sources, but they still contribute some riboflavin. A few highly enriched breakfast cereals contain 100 percent of the U.S. RDA in a single serving. The U.S. RDA for adults and children over four for riboflavin is 1.7 mg.

Food	Quantity	Percent of U.S. RDA
Beef liver	3 ounces	209.41
Product 19 breakfast cereal	1 ounce	100.00
Total breakfast cereal	1 ounce	100.00
Almonds; whole, shelled	1 cup	77.06
Milk shake, thick (made from mix)	10 ounces	38.24
Roe, baked or broiled	3 ounces	38.24
Avocado, raw (late summer, fall: Florida)	1 whole	35.88
Buttermilk, from skim milk	1 cup	25.88
Avocado, raw (mid-late winter: California)	1 whole	25.29
Wheaties breakfast cereal	1 ounce	24.70
Buttermilk, from whole milk	1 cup	24.12
Milk, whole or skim	1 cup	22.35
Cottage cheese	1 cup	20.00
Ice cream	1 cup	19.41
Yogurt (various types and flavors)	1 cup	18.82-31.17
Broccoli, cooked	1 cup	17.65
Spinach, cooked	1 cup	15.29
Asparagus, cooked	1 cup	12.94
Collards; leaves and stems, cooked	½ cup	11.76
Peanuts	1 cup	11.76

Riboflavin (Vitamin B_2)

GOOD SOURCES OF RIBOFLAVIN

Food	Quantity	Percent of U.S. RDA
Tuna	3 ounces	11.76
Pork chop, cooked	3½ ounces	11.18
Dandelion greens, cooked	½ cup	9.41
Beet greens, cooked	½ cup	8.82
Chicken	3 ounces	8.82
Egg	1 whole	8.82
Ground beef, cooked	3 ounces	8.82
Ham	3 ounces	8.82
Roast beef	3 ounces	8.82
Peas and beans; dried, cooked	1 cup	7.65
Cheese, natural and processed	1 ounce	6.47
Frankfurter	1	6.47
Brussels sprouts; frozen, cooked	3½ ounces	5.88
Green or snap beans	1 cup	5.88

Compiled from: CONSUMER GUIDE® magazine Nutrition Data Bank.

Riboflavin (Vitamin B$_2$)

RIBOFLAVIN CONTENT IN TWO DAILY DIETS

Typical Day's Diet for Woman (1,700 Calories)	Milligrams of Riboflavin
Breakfast	
4 ounces orange juice	0.01
1 ounce enriched corn flakes	0.42
1 slice enriched white toast	0.06
1 pat butter	none
1 cup 2-percent milk	0.40
Black coffee	none
Lunch	
Sandwich: 2 slices whole-wheat bread, 1 slice American cheese, 2 ounces boiled ham	0.21
1 cup skim milk	0.37
½ cup cole slaw	0.02
Dinner	
½ chicken breast, fried	0.17
1 medium baked potato	0.03
1 cup tossed green salad	0.03
½ cup peas, cooked	0.07
1 enriched dinner roll	0.06
2 pats butter	none
½ cup ice cream	0.16
Black coffee	none
Total	**2.01**
RDA	**1.20**

Compiled from: U.S.D.A. *Home and Garden Bulletin No. 72*, Washington, D.C., revised April, 1977.

Riboflavin (Vitamin B$_2$)

RIBOFLAVIN CONTENT IN TWO DAILY DIETS

Typical Day's Diet for Teenage Boy (3,000 Calories)	Milligrams of Riboflavin
Breakfast	
½ medium pink grapefruit	0.02
2 scrambled eggs	0.32
2 slices enriched white toast	0.12
1 pat butter	none
1 cup whole milk	0.40
Lunch	
1 cheeseburger	0.40
2 cups whole milk	0.80
10 large French-fried potatoes	0.01
1 medium banana	0.07
Dinner	
4 ounces round steak	0.25
1 cup green beans	0.12
1 cup mashed potatoes	0.11
Lettuce and tomato salad	0.03
2 slices enriched white bread	0.12
1 pat butter	none
1 cup whole milk	0.40
4 chocolate chip cookies	0.17
Snacks	
Cola drink	none
½ cup ice cream	0.16
¼ of 14-inch cheese pizza	0.06
Total	**3.56**
RDA	**1.80**

Compiled from: U.S.D.A. *Home and Garden Bulletin No. 72,* Washington, D.C., revised April, 1977.

Niacin

What do heart disease and schizophrenia have in common? The need for supplements containing large amounts of the B-complex vitamin known as niacin, some people say. However, when psychiatrists and experts in heart disease looked past the claims and searched for sound scientific evidence, they discovered that in practice, and even in theory, large doses of the vitamin are unwarranted. Only moderate doses are beneficial, and they are beneficial only for a particular disease, the disease that led investigators along the road to the discovery of this vitamin.

Niacin

History

The search for niacin, like that for other vitamins, was prompted by the quest for a cure for one disease. And like the search for other vitamins, the path that researchers followed to niacin took several wrong turns along the way.

In the early part of the 18th century, a disease characterized by red, rough skin began to appear in Europe. Almost 200 years later, the disease was still a scourge—at least for people in the southern United States.

The disease known as pellagra occurred in almost epidemic proportions in the South during the early 1900s. It appeared so often that many believed it was an infectious disease that spread from person to person; others thought it was caused by the eating of spoiled corn. Still others felt that it was spread by a type of fly because outbreaks of the malady were more severe in the spring when flies hatched.

Although pellagra was associated with corn-based diets, acceptance of the theory that it was caused by a dietary deficiency was slow in coming. One of the theory's first proponents, Dr. Joseph Goldberger, was convinced that the illness was caused by malnutrition. He began to experiment with various diets. First he added meat, milk, and eggs to the diet of children who suffered pellagra in a Mississippi orphanage and observed that the symptoms of the disease disappeared. Then in 1915 he conducted what has come to be considered a classic experiment in human nutrition.

For six months Goldberger ordered all the food that 11 volunteers from a Mississippi prison farm would eat. He selected for these volunteers the foods that were prevalent in areas hard hit by pellagra: corn, molasses, and fatty salt pork. At the end of the six months, seven of the 11 men showed symptoms of pellagra. When Goldberger changed their diets to include lean meat, milk, or yeast, the symptoms vanished. The experiment provided solid proof that pellagra was the result of a dietary deficiency.

Niacin

But some physicians still were not completely convinced. Many remained skeptical until 1937, when Conrad Elvehjem and his co-workers at the University of Wisconsin reported that dogs with pellagra-like symptoms could be cured with nicotinic acid. Soon, other investigators used nicotinic acid to cure pellagra in humans.

Food Sources of Niacin

In protein is a substance called tryptophan that can be turned into niacin in the body. But humans cannot create tryptophan; they must obtain it or the vitamin itself from food. Niacin is available in many foods. The best sources of niacin are foods that have a high content of protein: meat and eggs. Other good sources of niacin, such as milk, provide more tryptophan than niacin. (See the first table at the end of this chapter for the niacin content of some common foods. Also see the second table, which lists good food sources of the vitamin and the percent of the U.S. RDA for niacin provided by the foods.

Diets that include a variety of foods in the meat and dairy groups usually provide sufficient niacin. (See the third table at the end of this chapter for an estimate of the amount of niacin that can be provided in two typical menus.) Cereal-based diets, limited in quantity and variety, often are unsatisfactory or marginal when it comes to this vitamin.

Dietary Requirements for Niacin

Because the niacin value of a food or a diet depends on its content of pre-formed vitamin as well as tryptophan, the Food and Nutrition Board in 1968 prepared the Recommended Dietary Allowance (RDA) of the vitamin as milligram equivalents, which took into account pre-formed niacin and that available from tryptophan. The board estimated that 60 mg of tryptophan would yield 1 mg of the vitamin.

Niacin

In 1974, the board revised the RDA and expressed it as milligrams of the vitamin itself. Now the RDA for men and women allows 6.6 mg of niacin for every 1,000 calories and should be no less than 13 mg for women and 18 mg for men.

Function of Niacin

Niacin occurs in two forms—nicotinic acid and nicotinamide. Both forms are found naturally in foods. Nicotinic acid changes to nicotinamide in the body. There nicotinamide merges with other, more complex compounds to form coenzymes which are necessary for the metabolism of proteins, carbohydrates, and fats.

Deficiency of Niacin

Niacin deficiency, or pellagra, has been called the disease of the three Ds: dermatitis, diarrhea, and dementia. At first, pellagra causes weakness, loss of appetite, and some digestive disturbances. Soon the disease progresses. The skin becomes red and rough, but only on parts of the body exposed to sunlight, heat, or irritation. Also, the lining of the intestine might become suffused with blood and can develop ulcers, causing painful, serious diarrhea. In advanced cases, pellagra causes dementia or delirium.

If untreated, pellagra will severely damage the skin, the gastrointestinal tract, and the nervous system; and it can be fatal. Therefore, doctors must institute prompt and vigorous treatment. Important to consumers is what they can do to prevent the disease.

Experiments in which human subjects were fed varying amounts of niacin over an extended period of time indicate that a daily intake of from 9.2 to 13.3 mg of niacin will prevent the symptoms of deficiency. So the RDA of 13 mg for women and 18 mg for men will provide more than enough niacin to prevent pellagra.

Niacin

Therapeutic Uses of Niacin

A Food and Drug Administration Advisory Panel studying Vitamin and Mineral Drug Products for Over-the-Counter Human Use has found that 10 to 50 mg of niacin in a supplement can prevent deficiency with the higher dose being used by people who take drugs that interfere with the body's use of the vitamin, and by people such as chronic alcoholics who need more than the RDA for niacin. To treat deficiency 25 to 50 mg of niacin was recommended.[1]

Hazards and Toxicity of Niacin

At this point, scientists do not know how much nicotinamide, the form of niacin that is most often used in vitamin supplements, people can safely tolerate. However, doses of nicotinamide from 3 to 9 g a day have not caused adverse reactions.

In contrast, doses of nicotinic acid as low as 50 mg a day have dilated blood vessels and caused "flushing" due to the increased blood flow in expanded capillaries near the surface of the skin. They also have caused a burning sensation on the face and hands. Larger doses of nicotinic acid have induced nausea, vomiting, diarrhea, and skin rash, and they have activated dormant peptic ulcers. The response to large doses of nicotinic acid vary—apparently, some people are more sensitive to nicotinic acid than others.

Claims and Controversy

Large doses of nicotinic acid (3 g or more daily) lower the concentration of cholesterol in the blood. Since high blood levels of cholesterol are associated with heart disease, some investigators have proposed that such high doses might reduce the risk of heart attacks. In 1975 the Coronary Drug Project Research Group included nicotinic acid in a long-term test of the safety and effectiveness of

Niacin

certain drugs in the treatment of heart disease. For a number of months, 1,119 men who had had heart attacks received 3 g of nicotinic acid a day. These men were then compared with heart attack victims who received no drugs over the test period. The men who received nicotinic acid had fewer recurring heart attacks, but more gastrointestinal disturbances; more problems with irregular heartbeats (cardiac arrhythmias); and higher blood concentrations of the sugar glucose, and uric acid.

From this study, the researchers concluded that nicotinic acid might have a slight effect on the prevention of recurring heart attacks. However, because of the gastrointestinal problems, arrhythmias, and abnormal blood chemistry in the nicotinic acid group, they urged doctors to use "great care and caution" when prescribing nicotinic acid for treatment of heart disease.[2]

"Megavitamin therapy" and "orthomolecular treatment" are the popular names for the treatment of schizophrenia and other mental disorders with very large doses of vitamins. To evaluate the claims made by proponents of vitamin therapy, the American Psychiatric Association appointed a special task force in the early 1970s. After a careful review of the available evidence, the task force concluded that none of the claims could be confirmed, and that even the theory behind megavitamin treatment, especially treatment involving nicotinic acid, was suspect.[3]

Despite the lack of acceptable data to support them, these claims continue. The authors of *Supernutrition—Megavitamin Revolution* and *Psychodietitics* and other promoters of megavitamin therapy still advocate the use of large doses of niacin (3 to 9 g every day) and other vitamins in the treatment of schizophrenia and other mental disorders.[4,5] But this advice has no basis in scientific studies.

CONSUMER GUIDE® magazine Opinion

Advisors in this area warn that large doses of nicotinic acid

Niacin

have no apparent benefit, but do cause adverse effects in some people. To be safe, avoid nicotinic acid supplements.

Large doses of nicotinamide, the form most often used in vitamin supplements have not produced adverse or toxic effects, but nicotinamide should be used only according to a physician's advice to prevent or treat niacin deficiency.

Niacin

Type of vitamin: Water-soluble
Where stored in the body: The body does not store excess amounts of niacin.
History: Discovered in 1937
Food sources: Meats and eggs are the best sources; milk is a good source.
Recommended Dietary Allowance: 18 mg for men and 13 mg for women, based on 6.6 mg per 1,000 calories
Function: Niacin aids metabolism of proteins, carbohydrates, and fats.
Deficiency: Results in pellagra
Therapeutic uses: Physicians use vitamin supplements to treat or prevent niacin deficiency.
Hazards and toxicity: Large doses of nicotinic acid can cause flushing, nausea, vomiting, diarrhea, and skin rash; and can activate peptic ulcers in some people. Large doses of nicotinamide cause no adverse effects.
Claims and controversy: Large doses of nicotinic acid in the diet reduce the amount of cholesterol in the blood. Since high blood levels of cholesterol have been associated with heart disease, some investigators have suggested that nicotinic acid might decrease the risk of heart attack. A study of the safety and effectiveness of nicotinic acid showed that it might have a slight effect, but doctors must use it with caution because of known adverse reactions. Claims that supplements containing megadoses of niacin are beneficial in the treatment of mental disorders are unfounded.

Niacin

CONSUMER GUIDE® magazine's opinion: No adverse effects have been associated with large doses of nicotinamide in vitamin supplements, but nicotinamide should be used only when recommended by a physician to prevent or treat niacin deficiency. People who take drugs that interfere with niacin action, or people who need more than the RDA (chronic alcoholics, for example), may take supplements containing moderate doses of nicotinamide (50 mg). Large doses of nicotinic acid have caused some adverse effects in some people. So avoid using supplements of nicotinic acid, note the RDA, and eat a varied diet.

Niacin

NIACIN CONTENT OF COMMON FOODS

Food	Quantity	Milligrams of Niacin Pre-formed[1]	Milligrams of Niacin Equivalent[2]	Total Milligrams of Niacin
Milk Group				
Cheese; natural, processed	1 ounce	trace	1.2	1.2
Cottage cheese	1 cup	0.3	4.7	5.0
Ice cream	1 cup	0.1	0.8	0.9
Milk, whole or skim	1 cup	0.2	1.3	1.5
Yogurt	1 cup	0.3	2.0	2.3
Meat Group				
Egg	1 whole	trace	1.0	1.0
Beef liver	3 ounces	14.0	3.7	17.7
Bologna, 1-ounce slice	2 slices	4.6	1.0	5.6
Chicken	3 ounces	12.0	3.3	15.3
Dried peas, beans; cooked	1 cup	1.3	2.3	3.6
Frankfurter	1	1.4	1.0	2.4
Ground beef	3 ounces	4.6	3.8	8.4
Ham, baked	3 ounces	3.1	3.0	6.1
Roast beef	3 ounces	4.5	4.2	8.7
Cereal Group*				
Bread; white enriched, or whole-wheat	1 slice	0.8		

Niacin

Macaroni, noodles, spaghetti; enriched, cooked	1 cup	1.6
Oatmeal, cooked	1 cup	0.2
Ready-to-eat breakfast cereals, enriched		
Bran flakes, corn flakes, Wheaties	1 ounce each	5.0
King Vitaman	1 ounce	12.0
Product 19, Total	1 ounce each	20.0
Rice; enriched, cooked	1 cup	2.1
Fruit and Vegetable Group*		
Apple	1 medium	0.1
Asparagus, cooked	1 cup	0.9
Banana	1 medium	0.8
Carrot, raw	1 medium	0.4
Green or snap beans, cooked	1/2 cup	0.3
Orange	1 medium	0.5
Potato, baked	1 medium	2.7
Spinach, cooked	1/2 cup	0.5

1. Pre-formed niacin is that present as the vitamin itself.
2. Niacin equivalents refers to the niacin potentially available from the conversion in the body of the amino acid tryptophan to niacin.

* Cereal products, fruits, and vegetables have relatively low protein contents. Therefore, only the pre-formed niacin is shown for foods in these groups.

Compiled from: product labels and U.S.D.A. *Home and Garden Bulletin No. 72*, Washington, D.C., revised April, 1977.

Niacin

GOOD SOURCES OF NIACIN

This table lists a variety of foods that are good sources of niacin. The niacin value of a food depends on its content of pre-formed niacin (that present as the vitamin itself) as well as tryptophan, a substance in protein that can be turned into niacin in the body. The best sources of niacin have a high protein content: meat and eggs. Milk is another good source. Diets that include a variety of foods in the meat and dairy groups usually provide sufficient niacin.

The U.S. RDA for adults and children over four for niacin is 20 mg. In calculating the percentages of the U.S. RDA for niacin contained in the following foods, only the values for pre-formed niacin were considered. The percentages would be higher if the tryptophan contribution was included.

Food	Quantity	Percent of U.S. RDA
Peanut halves; roasted, salted	1 cup	123.50
Product 19 breakfast cereal	1 ounce	100.00
Total breakfast cereal	1 ounce	100.00
Beef liver	3 ounces	70.00
Tuna; canned in water (solids and liquid)	3½ ounces	66.50
Turkey, roasted	3½ ounces	49.00
Chicken liver, cooked	2 ounces	47.00
Chicken, roasted	3½ ounces	45.00
Salmon, broiled or baked	3 ounces	41.50
Beef round; bottom, broiled	4 ounces	32.50
Lamb chop, cooked	3½ ounces	32.50
Chicken; canned, boned	3½ ounces	27.50
Pork chop, cooked	3½ ounces	27.50
Ground beef	3 ounces	23.00
Roast beef	3 ounces	22.50
Ham, baked	3 ounces	15.50
Peanut butter	1 tablespoon	12.00
Frankfurter; all-beef, cooked	1	7.00

Niacin

GOOD SOURCES OF NIACIN

Food	Quantity	Percent of U.S. RDA
Dried peas, beans; cooked	1 cup	6.50
Cottage cheese, creamed	1 cup	1.50
Yogurt	1 cup	1.50
Milk, whole or skim	1 cup	1.00
Ice cream	1 cup	0.50
Cheese; natural and processed	1 ounce	*
Egg	1 whole	*

*This food contains only a trace of pre-formed niacin. The food's tryptophan content gives it value as a source of the vitamin.

Compiled from: CONSUMER GUIDE® magazine Nutrition Data Bank.

Niacin

NIACIN CONTENT IN TWO DAILY DIETS*

Typical Day's Diet for Woman (1,700 Calories)	Milligrams of Niacin
Breakfast	
4 ounces orange juice	0.4
1 ounce enriched corn flakes	5.0
1 slice enriched white toast	0.8
1 pat butter	none
1 cup 2-percent milk	0.2
Black coffee	none
Lunch	
Sandwich: 2 slices whole-wheat bread, 1 slice American cheese, 2 ounces boiled ham	2.2
1 cup skim milk	0.2
½ cup cole slaw	0.1
Dinner	
½ chicken breast, fried	11.6
1 medium baked potato	1.3
1 cup tossed green salad	0.2
½ cup peas, cooked	1.3
1 enriched dinner roll	0.9
2 pats butter	none
½ cup ice cream	0.5
Black coffee	none
Total	**24.7**
RDA	**13.0**

*Values for pre-formed niacin. Totals would be higher if tryptophan contribution were included.

Compiled from: U.S.D.A. *Home and Garden Bulletin No. 72,* Washington, D.C., revised April, 1977.

Niacin

NIACIN CONTENT IN TWO DAILY DIETS*

Typical Day's Diet for Teenage Boy (3,000 Calories)	Milligrams of Niacin
Breakfast	
½ medium pink grapefruit	0.2
2 scrambled eggs	none
2 slices enriched white toast	1.6
1 pat butter	none
1 cup whole milk	0.2
Lunch	
1 cheeseburger	6.4
2 cups whole milk	0.4
10 large French-fried potatoes	1.3
1 medium banana	0.8
Dinner	
4 ounces round steak	6.4
1 cup green beans	0.2
1 cup mashed potatoes	2.1
Lettuce and tomato salad	0.2
2 slices enriched white bread	1.6
1 pat butter	none
1 cup whole milk	0.2
4 chocolate chip cookies	0.9
Snacks	
Cola drink	none
½ cup ice cream	0.5
¼ of 14-inch cheese pizza	3.0
Total	**26.0**
RDA	**20.0**

*Values for pre-formed niacin. Totals would be higher if tryptophan contribution were included.

Compiled from: U.S.D.A. *Home and Garden Bulletin No. 72*, Washington, D.C., revised April, 1977.

Pantothenic Acid

Pantothenic acid is everywhere. It occurs in all living cells and can be found—at least to some extent—in all foods. Although the vitamin was discovered over 40 years ago, it has sparked little interest in nutritionists because a human deficiency is very rare. The vitamin is found in so many foods that dietary deficiency is unlikely. In fact, symptoms of vitamin deficiency occur in people only after long periods of food restriction. Nevertheless, some authors of popular books on nutrition blame pantothenic acid deficiency for arthritis, Addison's disease, and allergies. Conversely, others believe the vitamin can improve mental processes, get rid of gray hair, and ensure normal births.

Pantothenic Acid

History

Investigators were not looking for the cause of and cure for a specific human disease when they discovered pantothenic acid in the 1930s. They were looking for a substance that was necessary for growth of yeast. In the process researchers noted that diets lacking the isolated substance caused certain disorders in animals and that the symptoms of deficiency varied from species to species. Generally, however, animals fed diets without the substance had: a retarded growth rate; anemia; degenerated nerve tissue; decreased production of antibodies; ulcers; and they produced malformed offspring. The newly discovered vitamin was called pantothenic acid, derived from the Greek word *pantos,* meaning "everywhere."

Since many animal species proved to have a dietary requirement for pantothenic acid, scientists believed that people probably needed it, too. So in the 1950s investigators designed experiments to determine how a diet without pantothenic acid would affect human beings. In the experiments volunteers were fed a highly purified diet that lacked pantothenic acid but contained all other essential nutrients. After three or four weeks on this diet, the volunteers complained of weakness and an overall "unwell" feeling. One subject had burning cramps.

To accelerate and intensify the deficiency, a few volunteers received the pantothenic acid-deficient diet plus a compound that specifically interfered with the vitamin. These subjects developed symptoms faster than those in the other group, and they complained of insomnia, depression, gastrointestinal problems, leg cramps, and a burning sensation on the hands and feet. Like those in the original group, these subjects also had signs of reduced production of antibodies. For both groups of subjects, all symptoms disappeared after pantothenic acid was administered. Scientists concluded, therefore, that the experiments proved pantothenic acid was an essential nutrient for people.

Pantothenic Acid

Food Sources of Pantothenic Acid

All foods, regardless of their classification, contribute to the total daily intake of pantothenic acid, but organ meats (liver and kidney) and whole-grain cereals are the richest sources of the vitamin. Although cereal grains lose much of their natural pantothenic acid in the milling process, people who consume refined cereal products instead of whole-grain products still seem to get enough of the vitamin. At least at present, nutritionists are not urging food processors to restore the vitamin to refined cereal foods or to enrich ready-to-eat cereals with the vitamin. However, since the pantothenic acid status of the American people has not been extensively studied, there may be some need for pantothenic acid enrichment in the future. With continuous surveillance of the food supply, patterns of eating, and nutritional status of the American people, nutritionists eventually should be able to make more definite assessments of the need for pantothenic acid. (See the table at the end of this chapter for the pantothenic acid content of some common foods.)

Dietary Requirements for Pantothenic Acid

The Food and Nutrition Board has no Recommended Dietary Allowance (RDA) for pantothenic acid because there is not enough information on which to make a judgment of the daily dietary needs. Adult intakes of the vitamin range from 5 to 20 mg a day, and the Board believes that an intake of 5 to 10 mg probably is adequate for adults. In keeping with the Board's conclusion, the Food and Drug Administration includes in its list of U.S. RDAs (that is, the RDAs that appear on food labels) a value of 10 mg for pantothenic acid. Since pantothenic acid deficiency occurs only experimentally, there is no justification for taking more pantothenic acid than that supplied by an ordinary mixed diet.

Pantothenic Acid

Function of Pantothenic Acid

Pantothenic acid is an integral part of two complex biologic compounds which are needed to metabolize carbohydrates, fats, and proteins. The first of these—coenzyme A (CoA)—takes part in the energy-producing chain of reactions. The other—acyl carrier protein (ACP)—participates in the synthesis of fats.

Deficiency of Pantothenic Acid

Pantothenic acid deficiency is unlikely in people who eat an ordinary mixed diet. Symptoms of a marked deficiency have been seen only in experimental situations. Even then, severe symptoms occur only after subjects have been given a drug that interferes with the vitamin.

Therapeutic Uses of Pantothenic Acid

Pantothenic acid is not used to treat any health problem or condition other than its own deficiency.

Hazards and Toxicity of Pantothenic Acid

Studies on animals and humans have not shown any toxicity from large doses of pantothenic acid. However, massive doses (10 to 20 g a day) occasionally have caused diarrhea in human subjects.

Claims and Controversy

A common result of pantothenic acid deficiency in black rats is gray hair. Because lack of the vitamin caused the hair of black rats to turn gray, some investigators surmised that supplements of the vitamin may do just the opposite—prevent graying. But pantothenic acid does not prevent or reverse graying in people. To get rid of the gray, people must still depend on commercial tints and dyes.

Pantothenic Acid

Adelle Davis blamed pantothenic acid deficiency for arthritis, Addison's disease, and even allergies.[1] But only under extreme experimental situations has a marked deficiency been produced. So it is illogical to accuse pantothenic acid deficiency as the cause of these conditions.

Richard Passwater, Linda Clark, and Roger J. Williams, writers of popular books on nutrition, suggest that pantothenic acid may aid the treatment of arthritis.[2,3,4] Passwater claims, in addition, that it improves mental processes; and Williams suggests that the vitamin prevents birth defects. But these claims have been extrapolated from the findings of studies conducted on animals, and animal studies cannot always be directly applied to people. The value of any vitamin must be established by controlled experiments on human subjects.

CONSUMER GUIDE® magazine Opinion

A usual mixed diet provides more than enough pantothenic acid to meet the body's needs. Increased intakes of the vitamin provide no therapeutic benefit except to treat a rare case of deficiency.

Pantothenic Acid Summary

Type of vitamin: Water-soluble
Where stored in the body: The body does not store excess amounts of pantothenic acid.
History: Discovered in 1930s
Food sources: Organ meats (liver and kidney) and whole-grain cereals are the best sources.
Recommended Dietary Allowance: No RDA has been established. The usual mixed diets provide 5 to 20 mg, which is more than enough to meet the body's needs.
Function: Pantothenic acid is necessary for the metabolism of carbohydrates, fats, and proteins.
Deficiency: Pantothenic acid deficiency in people is

Pantothenic Acid

unlikely. It has occurred only in experimental situations or after periods of extreme food restriction.

Therapeutic uses: Pantothenic acid is used only to treat a rare deficiency of the vitamin.

Hazards and toxicity: Large doses of the vitamin in supplements have not caused any adverse effect, but doses in excess of 10 to 20 g a day have brought on an occasional bout of diarrhea.

Claims and controversy: Because pantothenic acid deficiency causes gray hair in animals, some investigators believed that extra amounts of the vitamin would do the opposite and prevent gray hair in humans. However, extra amounts of pantothenic acid have no effect on the graying process.

Pantothenic acid deficiency has been implicated as a cause of arthritis, Addison's disease, and allergies, but there is no evidence to support a connection between lack of the vitamin and these diseases.

Some authors claim that increased intakes of the vitamin will help cure arthritis, improve mental processes, and decrease the number and severity of birth defects. However, these claims are extrapolations of findings from animal studies; they have no proof in studies on humans.

CONSUMER GUIDE® magazine opinion: Body's needs met by usual mixed diet; supplements unnecessary.

Pantothenic Acid

PANTOTHENIC ACID CONTENT OF COMMON FOODS

Food	Quantity	Milligrams of Pantothenic Acid
Meat Group		
Beef liver, raw	3 ounces	6.55
Beef kidney, raw	3 ounces	3.27
Egg; fresh, raw	1 whole	0.80
Round steak	3 ounces	0.54
Ham, cured	3 ounces	0.48
Almonds; dried, shelled	3½ ounces	0.47
Salmon, canned	3 ounces	0.47
Ground beef	3 ounces	0.37
Pork chop; meat only, cooked	3 ounces	0.34
Liverwurst	1 ounce	0.22
Milk Group		
Milk, whole or skim	1 cup	0.84
Cottage cheese	1 cup	0.54
Ice cream	1 cup	0.53
Blue cheese	1 ounce	0.51
Cheddar cheese	1 ounce	0.14
Swiss cheese	1 ounce	0.10
Cereal Group		
100% Bran cereal	1 ounce	0.82
40% Bran Flakes cereal	1 ounce	0.25
Bread, whole-wheat	1 slice	0.19
Bread, rye	1 slice	0.13
Bread, white enriched	1 slice	0.11
Fruit and Vegetable Group		
Cauliflower, raw	3½ ounces	1.00
Grapefruit	½ medium	0.67
Corn, canned	1 cup	0.56
Banana	1 medium	0.45
Orange	1 medium	0.45
Asparagus, canned	1 cup	0.37
Tomato juice	4 ounces	0.28

Pantothenic Acid

PANTOTHENIC ACID CONTENT OF COMMON FOODS

Food	Quantity	Milligrams of Pantothenic Acid
Green beans, raw	3½ ounces	0.19
Apple, unpared	1 medium	0.15
Cabbage; shredded, raw	1 cup	0.14
Carrot, raw	1 medium	0.14

Compiled from: Orr, M.L., *Pantothenic Acid, Vitamin B_6 and Vitamin B_{12} in Foods,* Agricultural Research Service, U.S.D.A., Home Economics Research Report No. 36, Washington, D.C., 1969; and *Lessons on Meat,* National Live Stock and Meat Board, Chicago, 1976.

Vitamin B₆ (Pyridoxine)

Currently, nutritionists don't know whether the American people get enough vitamin B_6 or not. Although there is no evidence of widespread deficiency, some nutritionists believe that the usual intake of the vitamin is just barely enough. But until large-scale surveys of nutritional status directly assess vitamin B_6, nutritionists cannot say for certain whether people are getting their fair share of this B-complex vitamin.

History

The decade between 1930 and 1940 produced the discovery of one B vitamin after another. In 1933 it was

Vitamin B$_6$ (Pyridoxine)

riboflavin; a year later, thiamin. In 1937 it was niacin; then in 1939, vitamin B$_6$.

Vitamin B$_6$ is not one substance but three: pyridoxine, pyridoxamine, and pyridoxal. All three have the same biologic activity, and all three occur naturally in food. Plant foods generally are high in pyridoxine; pyridoxamine and pyridoxal are more common in animal foods. In one form or another, vitamin B$_6$ is found in all foods.

Food Sources of Vitamin B$_6$

Meats are excellent sources of vitamin B$_6$, and bananas, potatoes, and lima beans are other good food sources. Whole-grain cereal products provide the vitamin in good quantity, but their refined-grain counterparts do not offer as much. As is true for other B vitamins, much of the vitamin B$_6$ in grain is lost during milling. Milling removes the bran and germ of the grain—the sites of the B vitamins. Three B vitamins are restored in enriched white bread, wheat flour, and other cereal products. But vitamin B$_6$ is not.

Still, most people—even those who prefer refined over whole-grain foods—seem to get enough of the vitamin from other sources to prevent a full-scale deficiency. They may not be getting enough to prevent a so-called subclinical deficiency, however, a condition which occurs when the intake of a vitamin is just barely enough to meet the body's needs. It does not produce symptoms and, therefore, is difficult to detect.

So far, nutritionists in this country have not conducted extensive surveys to assess people's vitamin B$_6$ status. As they learn more about vitamin B$_6$ in the American diet, nutritionists will be in a better position to determine if people do get enough of the vitamin or if they need more. The Food and Nutrition Board has already proposed that refined cereal products be enriched with vitamin B$_6$.[1]

Already, some ready-to-eat cereals have been enriched with vitamin B$_6$. Corn flakes, Wheaties, Grape Nuts Flakes, and raisin bran breakfast cereals, for example, provide a

Vitamin B₆ (Pyridoxine)

quarter of the U.S. Recommended Daily Allowance (U.S. RDA) for the vitamin in a one-ounce serving. Other, more highly enriched cereals—Total, Product 19—provide 100 percent of the U.S. RDA in the same-size serving. (See the table at the end of this chapter for the vitamin B₆ content of some common foods.)

Dietary Requirements for Vitamin B₆

The requirement for vitamin B₆ depends in part on the amount of protein in the diet.[2] In one experiment, men who consumed 100 grams (g) of protein a day needed more vitamin B₆ than men who consumed 30 g of protein a day.[3] The Food and Nutrition Board recommends a daily vitamin B₆ intake of 2.0 mg for men and women, an amount sufficient to accommodate the high-protein diet that is common for most Americans. The RDA is raised to 2.5 mg a day for pregnant women because while women are pregnant they have increased needs for protein and for vitamin B₆. Women who take oral contraceptives containing estrogens may also need more vitamin B₆. However, at this time researchers are not sure if long-term use of oral contraceptives significantly changes nutritional requirements.[4] Evidence thus far suggests that women on oral contraceptives need more of certain vitamins, but it has not been proved that women on oral contraceptives need vitamin supplements.

Function of Vitamin B₆

Unlike the other B vitamins, vitamin B₆ is not directly involved in the production of energy. However, vitamin B₆ functions primarily in the metabolism of protein. In its active form as a coenzyme, vitamin B₆ helps metabolize amino acids, the products of protein digestion. It removes nitrogen from the amino acids to make them available as sources of energy. It also helps manufacture certain hormones, hemoglobin (the red, oxygen-carrying part of

Vitamin B$_6$ (Pyridoxine)

the blood), and other compounds that are important for normal function of the nerves and the brain.

Deficiency of Vitamin B$_6$

In experimental animals, vitamin B$_6$ deficiency causes skin inflammation, low concentration of hemoglobin in the blood, degeneration of nerve tissue, and convulsions. Some of these same symptoms were produced accidentally in infants in the 1950s when they were fed commercial liquid formula. Some 300 babies became irritable, and many had seizures because the formula contained too little vitamin B$_6$; it had been partially destroyed during manufacture of the formula. As soon as the babies received vitamin B$_6$, the symptoms disappeared.[5,6]

These babies are among the few people who have suffered vitamin B$_6$ deficiency. Since the vitamin is widely available in foods, dietary deficiency is rare. Vitamin B$_6$ deficiency however, has been induced in experimental situations.[7,8,9] In some experiments human volunteers were fed diets lacking in vitamin B$_6$. In other experimental situations the subjects also received an antivitamin, a compound which interfered with the action of the vitamin. Regardless of the way the deficiency was produced, people in the experiments developed certain symptoms. They had inflamed tongues and mouths, convulsions, and anemia. They became irritable and depressed, and they showed evidence of certain biochemical changes. The production of antibodies (the substances in the body that provide immunity to disease) was impaired. The excretion of two acids—xanthurenic acid and oxalic acid—increased. The amount of xanthurenic acid in the urine rose because there was not enough vitamin B$_6$ to completely metabolize the amino acid tryptophan and xanthurenic acid accumulated.

The reason for the rise in oxalic acid is not completely understood, but high concentrations of this acid in the urine are associated with kidney stones. This fact has

Vitamin B$_6$ (Pyridoxine)

been used to support the claim that vitamin B$_6$ deficiency may be at least partly responsible for kidney stones and that vitamin B$_6$ supplements may get rid of them. However, the Food and Drug Administration Advisory Panel on Vitamin and Mineral Drug Products for Over-the-Counter Human Use concluded that vitamin B$_6$ was not effective in the treatment of kidney stones.[10]

Therapeutic Uses of Vitamin B$_6$

Physicians prescribe vitamin B$_6$ in doses ranging from 7.5 to 25 mg a day to treat deficiency. They may recommend doses from 1.5 to 2.5 mg a day to prevent deficiency in people who have a disease that hinders the utilization of the vitamin.

Obstetricians commonly recommend multivitamin supplements that include vitamin B$_6$ for pregnant women. But most physicians do not recommend routine use of vitamin supplements for women who take oral contraceptives. For such women, there is still some question about whether or not the apparent increased need for vitamin B$_6$ is clinically significant and requires correction with a supplement of this vitamin.

Some drugs interfere with the action of vitamin B$_6$. For instance, while patients are taking the drug isoniazid (used in the treatment of tuberculosis) physicians prescribe 50 mg supplements of vitamin B$_6$. Likewise, physicians prescribe vitamin B$_6$ supplements while patients are taking penicillamine (used to clear the body of lead from lead poisoning and excess amounts of copper).[11]

Some hereditary disorders alter nutrient requirements. For example, a rare type of anemia is due to a biochemical defect in the body's hemoglobin-making mechanism. This type of anemia responds to vitamin B$_6$ supplements.

Hazards and Toxicity of Vitamin B$_6$

Large doses of vitamin B$_6$ do not cause any toxic

Vitamin B₆ (Pyridoxine)

reactions. Doses from 50 to 200 mg of the vitamin have been given daily for months with no discernible toxic effect. A few people have developed a temporary vitamin B₆ dependency after taking 200 to 300 mg doses of the vitamin for over a month. They experienced some unpleasant reactions, such as nervousness or tremulousness when they stopped taking such large doses of the vitamin. One report indicates that an infant may have an unusually high requirement for the vitamin if the mother takes high doses during pregnancy. Finally, large doses of vitamin B₆ interfere with the drug levodopa (L-Dopa), which is used in the treatment of Parkinson's disease.

Claims and Controversy

There have been reports that vitamin B₆ supplements relieve the morning sickness experienced during pregnancy. However, studies show that the vitamin cannot reduce nausea, and the Food and Drug Administration Advisory Panel on Vitamin and Mineral Drug Products for Over-the-Counter Human Use concluded that such claims are unproven.[10] (The FDA advisory panel came to the same conclusions for claims that vitamin B₆ could prevent or treat kidney stones.)

The late nutrition advocate, Adelle Davis, stated that "migraine headaches of long duration often clear up when vitamin B₆ is generously added to an otherwise adequate diet" and "at least fifty persons have told me that they have avoided painful hemorrhoid surgery by increasing their intake of vitamin B₆."[12] Davis provided no documentation for these vague and misleading statements, and no data are available to support them.

CONSUMER GUIDE® magazine Opinion

Although most people seem to get enough vitamin B₆ in their diets, nutritionists still do not have sufficient information to support or discredit this concept. At least for now,

Vitamin B$_6$ (Pyridoxine)

it's a good idea to stick to the RDA for this vitamin and to eat a variety of foods to attain it.

Vitamin B$_6$ Summary

Type of vitamin: Water-soluble
Where stored in the body: The body does not store excess amounts of vitamin B$_6$.
History: Discovered in 1939
Food sources: Vitamin B$_6$ is found in all foods; meats, whole-grain cereals, bananas, potatoes, and lima beans are the best sources.
Recommended Dietary Allowance: 2.0 mg for adults
Function: Vitamin B$_6$ acts in metabolism of protein, and helps produce certain hormones, hemoglobin (the red, oxygen-carrying part of the blood), and other compounds which are necessary for normal function of the brain and the nerves.
Deficiency: Dietary deficiency is rare. Experimentally induced deficiency has caused inflammation of mouth and tongue, irritability, depression, convulsions, anemia, and some biochemical changes.
Therapeutic uses: Physicians prescribe vitamin B$_6$ supplements to treat deficiency or to prevent it in people who are at high risk. Obstetricians commonly recommend multivitamin supplements that contain vitamin B$_6$ for pregnant women. Physicians prescribe vitamin supplements to patients who are taking drugs that interfere with the action of the vitamin. Finally, physicians use vitamin B$_6$ supplements to counteract a biochemical defect that is responsible for a rare type of anemia.
Hazards and toxicity: Doses of vitamin B$_6$ from 50 to 200 mg have not caused any adverse effects. Doses from 200 to 300 mg taken for over a month have produced a temporary dependency, and unpleasant reactions when people stop dosage. Large doses of the vitamin interfere with the drug levodopa (L-Dopa), used in the treatment of Parkinson's disease.

Vitamin B$_6$ (Pyridoxine)

Claims and controversy: Claims that vitamin B$_6$ supplements reduce the morning sickness of pregnancy have not been supported by controlled clinical studies. Available evidence shows that vitamin B$_6$ supplements have no effect in the prevention or treatment of kidney stones. Finally, no data have been found to confirm Adelle Davis's statements that vitamin B$_6$ will "clear up" migraine headaches and help people avoid painful hemorrhoid surgery.
CONSUMER GUIDE® magazine opinion: Until large-scale nutritional surveys determine the adequacy of vitamin B$_6$ in the American diet, stick to the RDA for this vitamin and eat different kinds of foods to meet it.

Vitamin B₆ (Pyridoxine)

VITAMIN B₆ CONTENT OF COMMON FOODS

Food	Quantity	Milligrams of Vitamin B₆
Meat Group		
Beef liver, raw	3 ounces	0.71
Chicken, uncooked	3 ounces	0.42
Pork chop; meat only, cooked	3 ounces	0.41
Ground beef, cooked	3 ounces	0.39
Round steak, cooked	3 ounces	0.39
Tuna, canned	3 ounces	0.36
Ham	3 ounces	0.30
Salmon, canned	3 ounces	0.25
Egg, fresh	1 whole	0.06
Cereal Group		
Ready-to-eat breakfast cereals (enriched)		
Special K, Total	1 ounce each	2.00
Corn flakes, Grape Nuts Flakes, raisin bran, Wheaties	1 ounce each	0.50
Bread, whole-wheat	1 slice	0.04
Bread, white enriched	1 slice	0.01
Milk Group		
Cottage cheese	1 cup	0.10
Milk, whole or skim	1 cup	0.10
Cheddar cheese	1 ounce	0.02
Fruit and Vegetable Group		
Banana	1 medium	0.89
Corn, canned	1 cup	0.51
Potato, uncooked	1 medium	0.25
Tomato juice	4 ounces	0.23
Green or snap beans, canned	1 cup	0.17

Vitamin B_6 (Pyridoxine)

VITAMIN B_6 CONTENT OF COMMON FOODS

Food	Quantity	Milligrams of Vitamin B_6
Lima beans, canned	1 cup	0.15
Spinach, canned	1 cup	0.13
Cabbage; chopped, raw	1 cup	0.11
Orange	1 medium	0.11
Grapefruit	½ medium	0.08
Carrot, raw	1 medium	0.07
Apple, unpared	1 medium	0.05
Potato chips	10 pieces	0.04

Compiled from: Orr, M. L., *Pantothenic Acid, Vitamin B_6 and Vitamin B_{12} in Foods,* Agricultural Research Service, U.S.D.A., Home Economics Research Report No. 36, Washington, D.C., 1969; and *Lessons on Meat,* National Live Stock and Meat Board, Chicago, 1976.

Biotin

"Caution! Egg whites may be hazardous to your health." No, the Surgeon General has not gone so far as to print that phrase on cartons of the popular food, and except for a man who was reported to live on six dozen raw eggs a week, no one is in any real danger. But almost 50 years ago, raw egg whites caused a real problem for experimental animals. And the cure for the animals' problem turned out to be an essential nutrient for people.

History

In the 1930s an investigator at the Lister Institute of Preventive Medicine in London, England, was experimenting with the diets of rats. After feeding the rodents raw egg

Biotin

whites for several weeks, he noticed that the animals developed an eczema-like skin condition, lost their hair, became paralyzed, and began to hemorrhage under the skin. Later, another team of investigators fed rats different foods to see which ones prevented or alleviated the "egg-white injury." Various kinds of foods were able to cure the rats' condition (dried yeast, milk, and egg yolk), and researchers zeroed in on them to discover what these foods held in common.

In 1940 Paul Gyorgy identified the substance common in these foods as a vitamin. At first, thinking the substance was a separate vitamin, he named it vitamin H. Soon scientists found that it was actually a member of the B-complex family, and they called it biotin.

Food Sources of Biotin

Biotin is a colorless, crystalline compound that occurs in just about every living cell, both plant and animal. Since some foods have proved to be especially good in reversing egg-white injury, they are considered to be better sources of the vitamin than other foods. Among these are organ meats such as liver and kidney.

Dietary Requirements for Biotin

People produce their own biotin by means of bacteria that live in the intestinal tract. Because of the difficulty of measuring how much biotin these bacteria actually make, nutritionists have been unable to establish how much biotin the body needs each day. However, they have found that ordinary mixed diets usually provide from 100 to 300 micrograms (μg) of biotin a day. This amount plus the amount produced by intestinal bacteria is enough.

Function of Biotin

Biotin acts as a coenzyme, or biologic catalyst, in several

Biotin

metabolic reactions. Some of these reactions are important for the manufacture of body fats; others are essential for the synthesis of glucose, a primary source of energy. In the synthesis of glucose, biotin-containing coenzymes metabolize proteins and create carbohydrates from non-carbohydrates. This process, called gluconeogenesis, sustains the body when the usual sources of carbohydrates are low (for instance, when a person is dieting) or absent (when a person is starving).

Deficiency of Biotin

Biotin deficiency is almost unheard of in man. It may, however, be induced experimentally.

When volunteers were fed large amounts of raw egg whites for several weeks, they developed biotin deficiency. The biotin deficiency occurred because raw egg whites contain a protein called avidin, which combines with the vitamin to form a biotin-avidin complex. In this complex biotin is bound so tightly that it cannot be released in the intestine and, therefore, cannot be absorbed by the body.

Experimentally induced biotin deficiency produces, in humans, symptoms similar to those caused by "egg-white injury" in rats: skin inflammation and loss of hair. It also brings on lethargy, loss of appetite, muscle pain, insomnia, and slight anemia. So biotin deficiency created experimentally is not really a lack of the vitamin but an inability to absorb it due to the presence of the raw egg white-contained protein, avidin. Since people do not eat raw egg whites to any great degree, and since the biotin produced by bacteria in the intestine usually make up for any dietary lack of the vitamin, biotin deficiency is no threat.

Therapeutic Uses of Biotin

A Food and Drug Administration Advisory Panel on Vitamin and Mineral Drug Products For Over-the-Counter Human Use concluded that there is no justification for

Biotin

including biotin in supplements designed to prevent or treat biotin deficiency since the deficiency simply does not occur.[1]

Hazards and Toxicity of Biotin

Large doses of biotin are not toxic, and they do not cause any adverse effects.

Claims and Controversy

Several investigators have reported that biotin helps reverse Leiner's disease—an oily skin rash on infants who are breast-fed by malnourished mothers. But other investigators have found that the disease was unaffected when infants were fed commercial formulas containing biotin. So far then, evidence of the role biotin plays in the treatment of Leiner's disease is conflicting. The Food and Drug Administration's advisory panel on over-the-counter vitamin-mineral drug products concluded that more research was needed before it could make any recommendation for the use of biotin for this disease. The panel did stress, however, that even if it found the vitamin to be valuable in the treatment of the disease, biotin should be given only under medical supervision.[1]

Richard Passwater, author of *Supernutrition—Megavitamin Revolution,* has speculated that biotin deficiency may be a factor in heart disease.[2] Since biotin deficiency isn't a human problem, it could hardly be a significant factor in heart disease.

Catharyn Elwood stated, "Biotin, another vitamin-B family member, is known as the mental-health vitamin."[3] In view of what has already been said about biotin deficiency in humans, it is illogical to expect a relationship between any disease, physical or mental, and a deficiency of the vitamin.

Biotin has been recommended as part of megavitamin therapy. But since biotin deficiency does not occur in

Biotin

people, there is no nutritionally sound basis for including the vitamin in supplements.

CONSUMER GUIDE® magazine Opinion

The biotin available in ordinary mixed diets plus that synthesized by intestinal bacteria is more than adequate to meet requirements. There is no reason to expect any therapeutic benefits from biotin in a supplement, and there is no need to eat certain foods in certain quantities to guard against biotin deficiency.

Biotin Summary

Type of vitamin: Water-soluble
Where stored in the body: The body does not store excess amounts of biotin.
History: Isolated in 1936
Food sources: Organ meats (liver and kidney) are considered to be the best sources.
Recommended Dietary Allowance: RDA not established; ordinary mixed diets provide 100 to 300 micrograms daily.
Function: As a coenzyme, biotin functions in the metabolism of carbohydrates, proteins, and fats.
Deficiency: Biotin deficiency does not occur in human beings unless induced by excessive indulgence in raw eggs.
Therapeutic uses: None demonstrated conclusively
Hazards and toxicity: No toxic or adverse reaction has been demonstrated.
Claims and controversy: Evidence that biotin is effective in the treatment of Leiner's disease is conflicting. More research is needed. Claims for biotin deficiency as a cause of any physical or mental disorder cannot be substantiated. There is no proof that biotin has any relationship to heart disease.
CONSUMER GUIDE® magazine opinion: Biotin deficien-

Biotin

cy does not occur in people. Consequently, there is no nutritionally sound reason for including the vitamin in supplements, no reason to expect any therapeutic benefit from biotin in supplements, and no need to eat certain foods in certain quantities to avoid biotin deficiency.

Folacin

Research leading to the discovery of folacin was closely related to the investigations which resulted in the discovery of vitamin B_{12}. These two vitamins work together in several important biological reactions. When the body lacks either folacin or vitamin B_{12} a characteristic type of anemia occurs. This is called megaloblastic or macrocytic anemia because the red blood cells are much larger than normal red cells.

History

As early as 1930, researcher Lucy Wills and her colleagues reported that yeast contained a substance which could cure the macrocytic anemia prevalent among the

Folacin

pregnant women in India, with whom they were working. It wasn't until the early 1940s, however, that the substance—folacin—was isolated and identified.

Folacin, folic acid, and folate all refer to the same B vitamin. In foods, most of the vitamin occurs in several different forms which together are called folacin. Folic acid is the simplest form of the vitamin. It is found in only small amounts in foods, but it is the form included in most vitamin supplements. The expression "folate activity" is often used to describe the actual biological potency or vitamin value of a food.

Food Sources of Folacin

Green, leafy vegetables such as asparagus, broccoli, and spinach are especially rich in folacin. Other vegetables, fruits, and organ meats (liver and kidney) are good sources. Milk and dairy products are only fair, and cereal foods generally are poor in folacin unless they are fortified. (See the first table at the end of this chapter for the folacin content of common foods.)

Dietary Requirements for Folacin

Studies indicate that the minimum adult requirement is 50 micrograms (μg) of folic acid each day. However, the Recommended Dietary Allowance (RDA) for folacin is eight times greater.

The Food and Nutrition Board recommends such a high RDA for two reasons. First, the minimum adult requirement of 50 μg is based on studies with pure folic acid. Pure folic acid is almost completely absorbed in the body, but other forms of the vitamin are not. About 75 percent of the folacin in an ordinary mixed diet comes from these other, less readily absorbed folates. Second, the available folacin in foods can be decreased by processing, handling, home preparation, and by storage. Nevertheless, most people can easily meet the RDAs.

Folacin

Although a person's actual intake of folacin is difficult to estimate, the Food and Nutrition Board says that an ordinary mixed diet can provide as much as 2,300 μg of the vitamin each day—much more than the Recommended Dietary Allowance for adults and adolescents (400 μg), for women who are breast-feeding (600 μg), and for pregnant women (800 μg).

Function of Folacin

Folacin functions as a coenzyme, or catalyst, in a number of biological reactions. One of the most important of these reactions is the synthesis of deoxyribonucleic acid (DNA). DNA carries the genes which determine the biological characteristics of an individual. When plants and animals grow, cells must divide and multiply. To do this a cell has to synthesize DNA, to double its supply, so that each of the two new cells has a full supply of the gene-containing material.

This function of folacin helps to explain why the vitamin is necessary for normal growth and development and why anemia occurs when there is not enough folacin. Large numbers of red blood cells have to be synthesized each day to replace the red cells which are normally destroyed. Synthesis of DNA is essential for this process.

Folacin is especially needed in any body tissue where new cells are constantly and rapidly being made. For example, millions of cells in the lining of the small intestine are destroyed each day and must be replaced.

Vitamin B_{12} is also necessary for synthesis of DNA. This explains why the same type of anemia (macrocytic) occurs when the body lacks either folacin or vitamin B_{12}.

Deficiency of Folacin

Folacin deficiency slows or stunts the growth of young animals. A deficiency of the vitamin causes a special type of anemia (macrocytic, megaloblastic) and severely dam-

Folacin

ages the lining of the small intestine. Thus people with folacin deficiency lose much of their ability to absorb nutrients from the foods they eat. Also folacin deficiency interferes with the production of white blood cells, which are important in combating infections.

Symptoms of folacin deficiency—sore, red, swollen tongue and inflamed intestines—may not appear for several months in adults on diets lacking in the vitamin. The body tends to hold on to its supply of folacin, although large excesses of the vitamin are rapidly excreted.

Folacin deficiency may develop within weeks, rather than months, in infants and children. Because they are growing rapidly, infants and children need proportionally more folacin than do adults.

Symptoms of folacin deficiency may occur rapidly in pregnant women also because they need more of the vitamin than when they are not pregnant. Pregnancy increases the need for folacin, because it is a time of rapid growth, of making new cells. Macrocytic anemia caused by folacin deficiency is quite prevalent among pregnant women subsisting on restricted diets such as those consumed by low-income populations in developing countries. Today folacin deficiency is probably the most common vitamin deficiency even in the developed countries of the Western world.

Physicians sometimes use compounds that interfere with folacin, called antagonists, as part of the treatment of cancer. Because folacin antagonists inhibit the action of the vitamin, they disturb the synthesis of DNA, thereby slowing down the growth of cancer cells. However, these drugs do not act against cancer cells only; they act on normal cells as well. Therefore, doctors must use them with extreme caution.

Other compounds that have a similar action against folacin are sometimes prescribed to treat psoriasis, to prevent malaria and convulsions, and to promote water loss from the body. Long-term use of folic acid antagonists may result in severe folacin deficiency. So doctors must

Folacin

weigh the benefits of use of the drugs against the risks of a folacin deficiency.

Therapeutic Uses of Folacin

A Food and Drug Administration advisory panel studying over-the-counter vitamin and mineral drug products has concluded that children over one year of age and adults could take supplements ranging from 0.10 to 0.40 mg (100 to 400 micrograms) a day to prevent folacin deficiency as long as the need for the supplements was determined by a physician. The panel suggested that pregnant women might need to take as much as 1.0 mg (1,000 micrograms) of folacin in supplements each day to prevent deficiency. However, the panel stressed that treatment of folacin deficiency could be managed safely only by a physician.[1]

Hazards and Toxicity of Folacin

Large amounts of folic acid are not toxic. Doses of 15 mg (about 40 times the RDA for adults) have not produced adverse effects. However, there is some evidence that greater doses may hinder the action of drugs taken by epileptics to prevent seizures. Further evaluation of folacin's effect on these drugs is needed.

The use of large doses of folacin is a hazard for persons with undiagnosed pernicious anemia. Macrocytic anemia is an early symptom of the disease. When this type of anemia is discovered, physicians conduct further tests to find out if pernicious anemia is the cause. However, large doses of folacin may prevent or correct macrocytic anemia, even in a patient with pernicious anemia. Diagnosis of the disease may be delayed, and serious, irreversible damage to the nervous system may occur. Folacin has no effect on the nerve damage of pernicious anemia. (See the chapter on vitamin B_{12} for more about pernicious anemia.)

As the final stage of his Supernutrition program, Richard

Folacin

Passwater recommends taking two high-potency vitamin-mineral supplements and two high-potency B-complex supplements each day.[2] Following Passwater's program could result in a folacin intake four times greater than the RDA. Although no toxicity has been associated with such high doses of the vitamin, these doses could delay the diagnosis of pernicious anemia, and the longer the delay, the more serious the damage to the nervous system.

Claims and Controversy

"The most glaring example of malnutrition by prescription occurs in women who take birth-control pills without supplementing their diet."[3] That's what the authors of *Psychodietitics* say. Although women who take oral contraceptives do have lower-than-usual blood levels of folacin and other vitamins, there has been no proof that these women have a serious vitamin deficiency. To date, the need for taking supplemental vitamins while on oral contraceptives has not been firmly established.[4]

In *Nutrition Against Disease,* Roger Williams tied folacin deficiency to some mental disorders.[5] Williams based his conclusions on studies which indicated that psychiatric patients had low concentrations of folacin in the blood. But such conclusions are faulty. The studies did not prove that a vitamin deficiency was actually present and did not show any causal relationship between the low blood levels of folacin and the psychiatric disorder. At the present time, there is no scientific basis for relating folacin deficiency to mental problems.

CONSUMER GUIDE® magazine Opinion

We do not recommend the use of folacin supplements. Supplements are needed to treat or prevent folacin deficiency. However, the treatment of such a deficiency should be left to a physician.

Folacin

Folacin Summary

Type of vitamin: Water-soluble
Where stored in the body: The body does not store excess amounts of folacin.
History: Discovered in early 1940s
Food sources: Green, leafy vegetables, other vegetables, organ meats (liver and kidney), fruits
Recommended Dietary Allowance: 400 micrograms (μg) for adults and adolescents; 600 μg for women who are breast-feeding; 800 μg for pregnant women
Function: Formation of red and white blood cells; production of gene-carrying material in the cells (DNA); growth promotion
Deficiency: Results in macrocytic anemia, stunted growth in young animals, damage to lining of small intestine causing poor absorption
Therapeutic uses: Physicians use supplements to treat or prevent folacin deficiency.
Hazards and toxicity: Large doses of supplemental folacin might interfere with the diagnosis of pernicious anemia.
Claims and controversy: Folacin deficiency has been implicated as the cause of some mental disorders. However, there is no solid proof of a connection between the two. Women who take oral contraceptives have lower-than-usual blood levels of folacin. Evidence does not show however, that these women have a vitamin deficiency serious enough to require treatment.
CONSUMER GUIDE® magazine opinion: Nonprescription vitamin supplements contain only 400 μg of folic acid per daily dose. Folic acid supplements are used to prevent or treat folacin deficiency. Only a physician can determine the need for supplements and prescribe adequate amounts of the vitamin.

Folacin

FOLACIN CONTENT OF COMMON FOODS

Food	Quantity	Micrograms of Folacin
Milk Group		
Cottage cheese	1 cup	29
Egg, hard-cooked	1 medium	22
Milk, whole	1 cup	12
Cheddar cheese	1 ounce	5
Meat Group		
Beef liver, cooked	3 ounces	123
Beans and nuts		
Pinto beans, cooked	1 cup	97
Almonds	½ cup	78
Peanuts	½ cup	75
Baked beans with tomato sauce	1 cup	61
Pecans	½ cup	48
Cashews	½ cup	47
Pork; lean, cooked	3 ounces	4
Beef; lean, cooked	3 ounces	3
Chicken; white meat, cooked	3 ounces	3
Ground beef, cooked	3 ounces	3
Cereal Group		
Ready-to-eat breakfast cereals (enriched)		
Product 19, Total	1 ounce each	400
King Vitaman	1 ounce	240
Corn flakes, Grape Nuts Flakes, raisin bran	1 ounce each	100
Bread, whole-wheat	1 slice	16
Bread, white enriched	1 slice	10
Fruit and Vegetable Group		
Banana	1 medium	118
Broccoli, cooked	1 medium spear	101

Folacin

FOLACIN CONTENT OF COMMON FOODS

Food	Quantity	Micrograms of Folacin
Spinach, cooked	½ cup	82
Orange	1 medium	65
Cabbage, raw	1 cup	62
Brussels sprouts, cooked	7 to 8	56
Tomato, raw	1 medium	53
Green or snap beans, cooked	½ cup	25
Potatoes, mashed	1 cup	21
Lettuce; leaf, raw	1 cup	20
Carrots, cooked	½ cup	18
Apple	1 medium	13
Grapefruit	½ medium	11
Potatoes, French-fried	10 pieces	11

Compiled from: product labels and Perloff, B.P. and Butrum, R.R., *Folacin in Selected Foods,* Journal of the American Dietetic Assoc. 70:161 (1977).

Vitamin B$_{12}$ (Cyanocobalamin)

Vitamin B$_{12}$ is unique. It differs from other vitamins, even those of the B-complex, in many ways. The vitamin has a chemical structure much more complex than that of any other vitamin. It is the only vitamin to contain an inorganic element as an integral part of its make-up. (There is one cobalt atom in each molecule of vitamin B$_{12}$.) Only microorganisms or bacteria can synthesize vitamin B$_{12}$. Plants and animals cannot make it.

Vitamin B$_{12}$ cannot be absorbed from the intestinal tract without the help of a substance which is made in the stomach—the intrinsic factor. The intrinsic factor combines with the vitamin B$_{12}$ released from food during digestion. It

Vitamin B$_{12}$ (Cyanocobalamin)

carries the vitamin to the lower part of the small intestine, where there are special receptor cells which the intrinsic factor recognizes and to which it attaches itself. The vitamin B$_{12}$ is released from its carrier and enters these cells to be absorbed into the body. Without the intrinsic factor vitamin B$_{12}$ will miss its connection with the receptor cells and will pass on out of the body.

Some people have an inherited disease known as pernicious anemia and cannot make the intrinsic factor. They cannot absorb vitamin B$_{12}$, even if there is plenty of the vitamin in their diets. Eventually they show symptoms of a vitamin B$_{12}$ deficiency.

History

The pursuit of vitamin B$_{12}$ began in 1926 when two investigators found that patients who ate almost a pound of raw liver a day were effectively relieved of pernicious anemia. But investigators did not know why. Scientists speculated that liver must contain some substance that prevents or cures the disorder, but they wondered why victims of pernicious anemia needed so much of it.

Scientist William Castle concluded that the liver contained an antipernicious anemia (APA) factor that is necessary to treat the anemia, but people who had the disease lacked an inside, or intrinsic factor necessary to use the APA. By eating about a pound of liver a day, these people could counteract the lack of the intrinsic factor and absorb enough APA.

For the next 20 years, scientists searched for the APA. Research was time consuming mainly because no experimental animals were suitable for the testing required, and extracts from liver had to be tried on humans instead. Scientists prepared extracts of liver and separated them into different fractions. Then each fraction was given to someone with pernicious anemia, and the researchers had to wait for a change to see which fraction contained the APA.

Vitamin B$_{12}$ (Cyanocobalamin)

Progress was slow until 1948, when an "experimental animal" was found—the microorganism, Lactobacillus lactis Dorner (LLD). Instead of testing liver extracts on people, researchers tested them on LLD. In less than a year two research groups found the answer. One research group in England and another in the United States isolated pure vitamin B$_{12}$ and extracted about 20 mg of the vitamin (also known as cyanocobalamin) from a ton of liver. Vitamin B$_{12}$ was the APA factor.

Food Sources of Vitamin B$_{12}$

Vitamin B$_{12}$ is present only in animal foods; plant foods furnish none of the vitamin unless fortified. Organ meats (liver and kidney), clams and oysters are the best sources of vitamin B$_{12}$. Other seafood, muscle meats, egg yolk and fermented cheeses such as Camembert and Limburger are good sources of vitamin B$_{12}$.

Bacteria that reside in the digestive tract of animals synthesize vitamin B$_{12}$. Most animals can absorb the vitamin made by the bacteria. However, in humans only the bacteria in the lower part of the intestinal tract synthesize vitamin B$_{12}$. The vitamin cannot be absorbed in this part of the tract. Consequently people must get their vitamin B$_{12}$ from foods.

The table at the end of this chapter shows the vitamin B$_{12}$ content of some common foods.

Dietary Requirements for Vitamin B$_{12}$

As far as vitamin B$_{12}$ is concerned, a little food goes a long way. The Recommended Dietary Allowance (RDA) is 3 micrograms (μg) for adults and 4 μg for pregnant and lactating women. You can easily exceed this RDA by simply eating a little liver or a bowl of cereal. Three ounces of liver provide more than 50 μg of the vitamin, and some ready-to-eat breakfast cereals fortified with the vitamin may have as much as 6 μg in a single serving.

Vitamin B$_{12}$ (Cyanocobalamin)

Function of Vitamin B$_{12}$

Vitamin B$_{12}$ and folacin are both essential for the synthesis of the gene-containing material of the cells, deoxyribonucleic acid (DNA). DNA carries the data bank for every living cell; that is, it delivers the messages that tell the cell how to function. Whenever a cell divides, DNA duplicates to pass on the messages from the parent to the offspring cell.

Some cells in the human body produce new generations more quickly than others; for example, red blood cells and cells that line the gastrointestinal tract. Each new generation of these rapidly reproducing cells needs its DNA complement. Without vitamin B$_{12}$, cells cannot divide and multiply.

Nerve fibers are covered by a sheath containing a substance called myelin. And the synthesis of myelin depends on vitamin B$_{12}$.

Deficiency of Vitamin B$_{12}$

When the supply of vitamin B$_{12}$ in the body is short, the production of red blood cells and of cells that line the gastrointestinal tract slows. A macrocytic anemia indistinguishable from that caused by folacin deficiency occurs. The damage to the intestinal tract is also similar to that of folacin deficiency. But unlike folacin deficiency, a lack of vitamin B$_{12}$ in the body also causes serious damage to the nervous system. The damage is often irreversible since nerve cells cannot be readily repaired or replaced.

Dietary deficiencies of vitamin B$_{12}$ are practically never seen. People usually get more than enough of the vitamin from eating animal food products. Further, the body tends to hold on to the vitamin B$_{12}$ absorbed from foods. Symptoms of vitamin B$_{12}$ deficiency do not appear in healthy adults for many months, even though the diet is lacking in the vitamin. Only strict vegetarians (people who eat no animal foods, not even milk or eggs) are likely to

Vitamin B_{12} (Cyanocobalamin)

develop symptoms of vitamin B_{12} deficiency.

Pernicious anemia is an inherited disease in which symptoms of vitamin B_{12} deficiency occur. But it is not caused by a lack of the vitamin in the diet. People with pernicious anemia cannot make the intrinsic factor, which is necessary for the absorption of vitamin B_{12}. Their diets contain the vitamin, but it cannot be absorbed.

The intrinsic factor is made in the stomach. Consequently, following surgical removal of the stomach, there is risk of developing vitamin B_{12} deficiency. Absorption of vitamin B_{12} may be reduced in regional ileitis (local inflammation of the small intestine). Regional ileitis damages the ileum, the part of the small intestine where the absorption of vitamin B_{12} takes place.

Therapeutic Uses of Vitamin B_{12}

Once it has been diagnosed, the treatment of pernicious anemia is vigorous. Physicians usually begin treatment by injecting the patient with 250 µg of vitamin B_{12} once or twice a week for several months, then once or twice a month for a year.

Once the progress of the disease has been arrested, physicians start their patients on maintenance therapy. People with pernicious anemia have permanently lost the ability to absorb vitamin B_{12}. To provide enough vitamin B_{12} for DNA and myelin synthesis, physicians administer an injection of 100 µg of vitamin B_{12} each month for the rest of the patient's life.

To effectively reverse pernicious anemia, vitamin B_{12} must be injected. Serious nervous system damage may result if people take oral vitamin supplements instead of seeing their physician for injections. Also, oral vitamin B_{12} supplements should be avoided by patients with regional ileitis or following surgical removal of the stomach. Oral vitamin B_{12} supplements are safe and effective only to prevent or to treat a dietary deficiency.

Since dietary deficiency is rare, oral vitamin B_{12} supple-

Vitamin B_{12} (Cyanocobalamin)

ments are appropriate only for strict vegetarians. People following such diet regimens apparently get at least a little vitamin B_{12} through bacterial "contamination" of food, but they still should supplement their diet with the vitamin. Strict vegetarians, especially mothers-to-be and nursing mothers, should take 25 to 50 µg of vitamin B_{12} once or twice a week. Lacto-ovo-vegetarians, people who eat no meat but do eat eggs and drink milk, have no need for vitamin B_{12} supplements.

Hazards and Toxicity of Vitamin B_{12}

Even when used in large amounts for several years, vitamin B_{12} does not cause toxicity or any apparent adverse effect, but use of oral supplements should be guarded. Serious damage to the nervous system can result when people with undiagnosed pernicious anemia take oral supplements. To correct the anemia, vitamin B_{12} must be injected.

Claims and Controversy

When referring to vitamin B_{12}, the name "antianemia vitamin" often is bandied about. But vitamin B_{12} is used to treat only pernicious anemia. It is not effective in the treatment of other, more common anemias such as those due to iron or folacin deficiencies. So, "antianemia vitamin" is a misnomer.

In *Let's Eat Right To Keep Fit,* Adelle Davis noted that "if the diet of the person lacking vitamin B_{12} is otherwise adequate . . . he does not develop anemia. Pernicious anemia results from simultaneous deficiencies of both vitamin B_{12} and folic acid. . . ."[1] This statement is totally inconsistent with what is known about the cause of pernicious anemia and the nature of vitamin B_{12} deficiency. The real cause of pernicious anemia is the inability to synthesize the intrinsic factor; dietary deficiency is rare. So, claiming that simultaneous deficiencies of vitamin B_{12}

Vitamin B_{12} (Cyanocobalamin)

and folic acid are the cause of pernicious anemia is misleading and dangerous.

In a brochure the Windmill Natural Vitamin Company states that vitamin B_{12} increases the production of red blood cells, provides energy, and improves mental health. Yet none of these claims is true. First, vitamin B_{12} is essential for the manufacture of red blood cells, but excess amounts of the vitamin will not cause production of excess numbers of red blood cells. If so, people who took large doses of the vitamin soon would have blood vessels clogged with cells. Second, like any vitamin, B_{12} is not—by itself—a source of energy. Finally, although there is no evidence to substantiate the view that vitamin B_{12} aids mental health, large amounts of the vitamin have been included in megavitamin therapies for just that reason. As Dr. Victor Herbert concluded after a recent review of vitamin B_{12}: "Unfortunately, [vitamin B_{12}] is . . . used by megahustlers to make megabucks selling oral tablets containing megaquantities of the vitamin for a wide range of claimed but nonexistent effects."[2]

CONSUMER GUIDE® magazine Opinion

Vitamin B_{12} supplements are unnecessary except for strict vegetarians and for sufferers of pernicious anemia who, under a physician's care, should receive supplemental injections.

Vitamin B_{12} Summary

Type of vitamin: Water-soluble
Where stored in the body: The liver stores small amounts of Vitamin B_{12}.
History: Discovered in 1948
Food sources: Meats, seafood, egg yolk, fermented cheeses. Vitamin B_{12} is only found in animal foods.
Recommended Dietary Allowance: 3 µg for adults; 4 µg for pregnant women.

Vitamin B_{12} (Cyanocobalamin)

Function: To aid synthesis of the gene-containing material of cells—deoxyribonucleic acid (DNA)—and the substance that covers nerve cells (myelin)

Deficiency: Pernicious anemia results from inability to absorb vitamin B_{12}. Dietary deficiency is rare.

Therapeutic uses: Physicians use vitamin B_{12} injections to treat pernicious anemia. Strict vegetarians probably should take 25 to 50 µg of vitamin B_{12} in supplement form once or twice a week to prevent dietary deficiency. Any disease or condition which hinders vitamin B_{12} absorption is treated with B_{12} injections to prevent deficiency.

Hazards and toxicity: No toxic or adverse reactions have been known to occur following large doses of vitamin B_{12}, but oral vitamin supplements are considered to be safe and effective only to prevent dietary deficiency in strict vegetarians. Serious nervous system damage may occur if people use oral vitamin B_{12} supplements to treat pernicious anemia instead of receiving injections.

Claims and controversy: Injections of vitamin B_{12} correct pernicious anemia only. They have no effect on other, more common types of anemia. The belief that pernicious anemia arises from vitamin B_{12} and folic acid deficiencies is erroneous. Pernicious anemia is due to the body's inability to absorb the vitamin. Though vitamin B_{12} is necessary for the production of red blood cells, more vitamin B_{12} will not generate excess red blood cells. Like other vitamins, vitamin B_{12} is not by itself a source of energy. Though megadoses of the vitamin have been advocated to ensure mental health, there is no evidence to support their use for this.

CONSUMER GUIDE® magazine opinion: The RDA for vitamin B_{12} is small and can be met easily by most diets. However, strict vegetarians probably should take a vitamin B_{12} supplement once or twice a week. People who suffer from pernicious anemia should not try to treat their condition on their own but must see a physician regularly for therapy to prevent damage to nerves.

Vitamin B_{12} (Cyanocobalamin)

VITAMIN B_{12} CONTENT OF COMMON FOODS

Food	Quantity	Micrograms of Vitamin B_{12}
Beef liver, raw	3 ounces	68.0
Beef kidney, raw	3 ounces	26.3
Sardines, canned	3 ounces	8.5
Liverwurst	1 ounce	3.9
Cottage cheese	1 cup	2.5
Tuna, canned	3 ounces	1.9
Round steak, cooked	3 ounces	1.4
Egg, fresh	1 whole	1.0
Ground beef, cooked	3 ounces	1.0
Milk, whole or skim	1 cup	1.0
Frankfurter, raw	1	0.6
Pork, cooked	3 ounces	0.5
Cheddar cheese	1 ounce	0.3

Compiled from: Orr, M.L.: *Pantothenic Acid, Vitamin B_6 and Vitamin B_{12} in Foods,* Agricultural Research Service, U.S.D.A., Home Economics Research Report No. 36, Washington, D.C., 1969; and *Lessons on Meat,* National Live Stock and Meat Board, Chicago, 1976.

Vitamin C (Ascorbic Acid)

When asked the first thing that comes into their heads when they hear "vitamin C," many people respond "Linus Pauling" or "the common cold." Although they might not agree with him, most people have heard of Pauling and his book *Vitamin C and the Common Cold*.[1]

In his 1970 book, Pauling espoused megadoses of vitamin C to reduce the frequency and severity of colds. The book triggered a sales boom for vitamin C. It also prompted nutritionists to begin a series of carefully designed studies of the vitamin. Today, some people still swear by vitamin C, but nutritionists have found little proof of its effectiveness against the common cold.

Vitamin C (Ascorbic Acid)

History

The story of vitamin C begins centuries before the discovery of the vitamin, with accounts of a disease called scurvy.

Scurvy—an ailment characterized by muscle weakness, lethargy, and bleeding under the skin—has been rampant around the world throughout the centuries. Documents written before the birth of Christ describe the disease. Ships' logs tell of its widespread occurrence among sailors in the 16th century. History books report that scurvy was a common problem among the troops during the American Civil War. And records of Antarctic explorers recount how Captain Robert Scott and his team succumbed to the malady in 1912.

Almost as old as the reports of the disease are the reports of successful ways of treating it. Over the centuries, references were made to the curative properties of green salads, fruits, vegetables, pickled cabbage, small onions, and an ale made of wormwood, horseradish, mustard seed and the like. In the 1530s, the French explorer Jacques Cartier told how Newfoundland Indians cured the disease by giving his men an extract prepared from the green shoots of an evergreen tree.

The disease was still the "scourge of the navy" 200 years later when the British physician James Lind began an experiment that singled out, once and for all, a cure for scurvy.[2] Believing that acidic materials would relieve the illness, Lind tried six different substances on six groups of men suffering with scurvy. He gave all the men the standard shipboard diet, but to a pair of men in each of the six groups he gave a different test substance. One pair received a solution of sulfuric acid each day; another, cider; and a third, sea water. The fourth group received vinegar, and the fifth took a combination of garlic, mustard seed, balsam of Peru, and gum myrrh daily. The last group received two oranges and a lemon each day.

Lind found that the men who had eaten the citrus fruit

Vitamin C (Ascorbic Acid)

improved rapidly; one was able to return to duty after only six days. The sailors who drank the cider showed slight improvement after two weeks, but those who had received the other test substances did not improve. Although Lind soon published the results of his experiment, 50 years passed before the British navy finally added lemon juice to its sailors' diets to prevent scurvy.

The discovery of the cure for scurvy marked the end of one chapter in the story of vitamin C. The next chapter ended in 1932 with the isolation of the vitamin by C. G. King and W. A. Waugh at the University of Pittsburgh and by Albert Szent-Gyorgyi in Hungary.[3,4]

At the time Szent-Gyorgyi isolated the vitamin, he knew little of its chemical makeup. He knew only that it exhibited some similarities to sugar. He first proposed that the vitamin be given the name ignose, from the Latin *ignosco* for "I do not know" and *ose,* the suffix applied to sugars. The editor of a British scientific journal would not accept the name, so Szent-Gyorgyi suggested an alternative: godnose. When Szent-Gyorgyi's article was finally published in the journal, the vitamin carried the name hexuronic acid. Later the name was changed to ascorbic (meaning "without scurvy") acid.

Food Sources of Vitamin C

Most mammals can manufacture all the vitamin C they need, but man cannot, so he must turn to foods. The best foods to turn to are fruits and vegetables.

The citrus fruits—oranges, lemons, limes, grapefruit—are excellent sources of the vitamin. Strawberries, cantaloupe, and raw peppers supply large amounts of it. Milk and milk products provide little vitamin C, but breast milk contains enough ascorbic acid to meet the needs of a nursing infant during the first few months of life. Meats, other than organ meats (liver and kidney), have no vitamin C; nor do unfortified cereal products.

Many fruit-flavored drinks and drink mixes are fortified

Vitamin C (Ascorbic Acid)

with ascorbic acid, and the amount of vitamin C provided in a few ounces sometimes exceeds the Recommended Dietary Allowance (RDA). (See the first table at the end of this chapter for the ascorbic acid content of many fortified drinks and drink mixes, as well as the vitamin content of other common foods.)

Vitamin C is often added to foods as a preservative because it interferes with oxidation. It is added to some cured meats because it inhibits the formation of nitrosoamines, compounds that have caused cancer in experimental animals. The significance of this action of vitamin C to human health is not known.

More than any other vitamin, vitamin C is subject to destruction. The ascorbic acid value of foods decreases rapidly during transport, processing, storage, and preparation. Even if fresh produce and fruit drinks are refrigerated and protected from the air by packaging, the vitamin gradually deteriorates. Even if fruits and vegetables are quick-frozen and stored, they slowly lose their vitamin activity. The best bet when it comes to vitamin C is fresh fruit and vegetables. Generally, they have a higher ascorbic acid content than their processed or cooked counterparts.

Dietary Requirements for Vitamin C

Clinicians have found that a daily intake of 10 mg of ascorbic acid will cure or prevent scurvy. This amount, however, is not enough to maintain a normal concentration of the vitamin in the blood or in the body. In keeping with the philosophy that good nutrition means more than simply preventing vitamin deficiency, the Food and Nutrition Board recommends a daily intake of 45 mg of the vitamin for adults. This RDA approximates the amount of the vitamin that is needed to maintain normal levels of ascorbic acid in the blood and tissues.

Some nutritionists believe that the RDA should be increased by 50 to 100 percent. They think the RDA does

Vitamin C (Ascorbic Acid)

not provide enough to ensure complete tissue saturation. An individual easily could meet a higher RDA. For example, in a half cup of cooked broccoli is 70 mg of ascorbic acid, enough to meet an allowance 50 percent higher than the current RDA. A half cantaloupe contains 90 mg of ascorbic acid, enough to double today's Recommended Dietary Allowance. (See the second table at the end of this chapter for a list of good food sources of vitamin C and the percent of the U.S. RDA they provide.

Function of Vitamin C

Little is known about how vitamin C works in the body. It may act as a coenzyme, and it appears to be a factor in a number of oxidation-reduction reactions. As an antioxidant, vitamin C protects such oxygen-sensitive compounds as vitamins A and E, and polyunsaturated fatty acids.

Although scientists do not know exactly how vitamin C works, they do know something about what it does. Vitamin C helps the body synthesize collagen, the connective tissue that holds the body's cells and tissues together. It promotes normal development of bones and teeth; it plays a role in the metabolism of some amino acids, the compounds that make up protein molecules; and it is involved in the synthesis of certain hormones and other compounds that take part in the transfer of nerve impulses.

Scientists have suggested other functions for the vitamin: It may participate in the metabolism of fats and cholesterol, and it seems to affect the formation of blood cells and blood clotting. There still is much to be learned about the function of vitamin C.

Deficiency of Vitamin C

Vitamin C deficiency, or scurvy, causes muscle weakness, swollen and bleeding gums, loss of teeth, and bleeding under the skin. People who have scurvy tire easily, and

Vitamin C (Ascorbic Acid)

they may become depressed. Usually, a dietary lack does not cause signs of deficiency for two to three months. During that period, there is a marked reduction in the concentration of the vitamin in the blood. Because vitamin C is needed for the synthesis of collagen, a person who is deficient in vitamin C and wounds himself will heal slowly.

Therapeutic Uses of Vitamin C

Physicians prescribe doses of ascorbic acid to prevent or treat deficiency. Therapeutic doses of vitamin C have not been proved beneficial in the treatment of other conditions.

Hazards and Toxicity of Vitamin C

Large, single doses of vitamin C are not toxic. Large doses of the vitamin taken every day for more than a year cause no serious adverse effects in most people. A few people have complained of abdominal discomfort, diarrhea, and cramps. These side effects apparently occur in only a small percentage of people who use vitamin C supplements. Also, people who have a hereditary disorder that makes them prone to kidney stones may develop them faster when taking megadoses of vitamin C.

After taking massive doses of the vitamin for an extended period of time, people might not develop any toxic reactions, but their bodies might become conditioned to the increased intake; that is, their bodies can become used to the excessive amounts of the vitamin. When they stop taking ascorbic acid supplements, their bodies' demands for the vitamin are not met by the normal, dietary intake, and they develop symptoms of vitamin C deficiency. Similar to this effect is the development of scurvy among infants whose mothers took large amounts of the vitamin during pregnancy. Apparently the infants have an increased requirement for ascorbic acid due to their exposure to extra amounts of the vitamin from their mothers.

Vitamin C (Ascorbic Acid)

Megadoses of vitamin C can interfere with certain laboratory tests. For example, some people who take large amounts of ascorbic acid exhibit what appear to be signs of diabetes in their urine when, in fact, they do not have that disease; or a blood test may fail to indicate liver disease when it is present. And large doses of the vitamin can counteract the effect of drugs used to dissolve blood clots.

(See reference numbers 5 and 6 for sources of this section's information.)

Claims and Controversy

Promoters of megavitamin therapy recommend massive doses of ascorbic acid along with large amounts of other vitamins to prevent or to treat a variety of diseases, both physical and mental. For example, Richard Passwater suggests 3 grams (g) of ascorbic acid a day as part of his Supernutrition program to prevent a variety of diseases.[7] The authors of *Psychodietetics* say that ascorbic acid is one of the vitamins that can prevent senility.[8] And they report that 1 to 12 g of ascorbic acid a day can be used as part of the treatment of schizophrenia. However, the Food and Drug Administration Advisory Panel on Vitamin and Mineral Drug Products for Over-the-Counter Human Use concluded that controlled clinical studies do not support the claims for using vitamin C to treat atherosclerosis (hardening of the arteries), allergy, mental illnesses including schizophrenia, corneal ulcers, thrombosis (blood clots), or pressure sores.[9]

People who have a vitamin C deficiency are susceptible to infection, so many researchers have thought that ascorbic acid might provide some resistance to infection. But scientists have not been able to demonstrate conclusively that supplemental vitamin C provides such protection.

Some advertisements suggest that cigarette smokers need more vitamin C than nonsmokers. While it is true

Vitamin C (Ascorbic Acid)

that, on the average, the concentration of the vitamin in the blood is lower in smokers than in nonsmokers, the concentration is still within the normal range. Smokers who eat an ordinary mixed diet need not take vitamin C supplements.

Since 1970, nutritionists have been conducting research designed to prove or disprove Linus Pauling's claims that megadoses of vitamin C could prevent or treat the common cold. In his book, Pauling cited the results of some studies that were not acceptable from a scientific point of view.

Some of these studies did not compare similar groups of people. That is, the volunteers who received vitamin C were not always matched according to age, sex, occupation, place of residence, or life-style with volunteers used as a control group. Nor did all of the studies rule out the placebo effect. It has been well established in medicine that the very act of treatment seems to have a positive psychologic effect on the recipient of that treatment. For example, when a completely inert substance is given to a patient, he may observe some improvement if he believes the substance is therapeutic. So controlled clinical trials must provide to the control group a placebo, or a preparation that is identical in appearance with the active drug given to the experimental group. Then the true effects of the drugs can be separated from the psychologic effects of the placebo. And the studies Pauling cited were not always double-blind. In a double-blind study, neither the subjects nor the investigators know in advance whether a subject is receiving the active drug or a placebo.

Since the publication of *Vitamin C and the Common Cold,* a number of double-blind studies have been conducted. In these studies, large doses of vitamin C were given to one group of volunteers, and placebos were given to another, similar group of volunteers. In some but not all of the studies, large amounts of ascorbic acid showed a slight beneficial effect in reducing the severity of colds, apparently because the vitamin acted as an antihistamine.

Vitamin C (Ascorbic Acid)

For the most part, however, the studies did not prove that large amounts of the vitamin prevented a cold.[10-16]

Most of the recent trials of vitamin C therapy have been complicated by numerous factors beyond the control of the researchers. First, large-scale field trials obtained data by asking participants about their colds: the occurrence, severity, and duration. Such data are subject to more variation and error than are data obtained from objective, clinical evaluations. The trials also were affected by the nature of colds: A cold generally lasts for only a few days, and it often goes away without any treatment at all. Furthermore, people differ in their definitions of what constitutes a cold.

Despite those problems, most of the studies that followed the publication of Pauling's book were reasonably well designed. The Department of Drugs of the American Medical Association concluded: "[the studies provided] little convincing evidence to support claims of clinically important efficacy. Until such time as pharmacologic doses of ascorbic acid have been shown to have obvious, important clinical value in the prevention and treatment of the common cold, and to be safe in the large varied population, we cannot advocate its unrestricted use for such purposes."[17]

CONSUMER GUIDE® magazine Opinion

To meet your body's needs, amounts of vitamin C approximating the RDA should be taken.

Vitamin C Summary

Type of vitamin: Water-soluble
Where stored in the body: The body does not store excess amounts of Vitamin C.
History: Discovered in 1932
Food sources: Citrus fruits—oranges, lemons, limes, grapefruit—are excellent sources of the vitamin. Straw-

Vitamin C (Ascorbic Acid)

berries, cantaloupe, and raw peppers are good sources.
Recommended Dietary Allowance: 45 mg for adults
Function: Ascorbic acid helps the body synthesize the connective tissue that holds the cells and tissues together; promotes normal development of bones and teeth; plays a role in the metabolism of amino acids (parts of protein molecules); and helps manufacture certain hormones and other compounds that take part in the transfer of nerve impulses.
Deficiency: Results in scurvy
Therapeutic uses: To prevent and treat ascorbic acid deficiency
Hazards and toxicity: A few people have complained of abdominal discomfort, diarrhea, and cramps after taking large doses of ascorbic acid. However, the effects apparently occur in only a small percentage of the people who take massive doses of vitamin C. People who have a hereditary disorder that makes them prone to kidney stones might develop stones faster when taking large doses of vitamin C. After taking massive doses of the vitamin for an extended period of time, people may become conditioned to the increased intake. They may develop symptoms of deficiency when they stop ingesting the vitamin because their bodies have become used to the large doses. Megadoses of vitamin C may interfere with tests of urine and blood, and cause errors in the diagnosis of disease. Large doses of the vitamin may counteract the effect of drugs used to dissolve blood clots.
Claims and controversy: Promoters of megavitamin therapy recommend massive doses of ascorbic acid to treat a variety of physical and mental diseases. However, the FDA advisory panel on over-the-counter vitamin-mineral drug products concluded that vitamin C was not effective in the treatment of atherosclerosis (hardening of the arteries), allergies, mental illnesses including schizophrenia, corneal ulcers, thrombosis (blood clots), and pressure sores. People with vitamin C

Vitamin C (Ascorbic Acid)

deficiency are susceptible to infection. For them, ascorbic acid supplements improve resistance to infection. For people who do not have vitamin C deficiency, ascorbic acid supplements have had no effect on the body's ability to resist infection. The concentration of vitamin C in the blood of smokers is lower than that of nonsmokers, but it still is within the normal range. Smokers who eat an adequate diet do not need vitamin C supplements. Tests have not shown that vitamin C has any clinical value in the prevention or treatment of the common cold.

CONSUMER GUIDE® magazine opinion: Amounts of vitamin C approximating the RDA should provide enough to maintain a normal concentration in the blood and the body. More than this amount of the vitamin has not been shown to be effective in the treatment of physical or mental disorders.

Vitamin C (Ascorbic Acid)

VITAMIN C CONTENT OF COMMON FOODS*

Food	Quantity	Milligrams of Vitamin C
Fruits		
Cantaloupe	½ melon	90
Orange	1 medium	66
Orange juice; frozen, diluted	4 ounces	60
Grapefruit	½ medium	44
Strawberries, fresh	½ cup	44
Banana	1 medium	12
Apple	1 medium	6
Apricots, canned	½ cup	5
Vegetables		
Broccoli; chopped, cooked	½ cup	70
Cauliflower; chopped, raw	½ cup	45
Potato, baked	1 medium	31
Tomato, raw	1 medium	28
Tomato juice, canned	4 ounces	20
Asparagus, cooked	½ cup	19
Cabbage; shredded, raw	½ cup	17
Potato, mashed	½ cup	10
Green or snap beans, cooked	½ cup	8
Carrot, raw	1 medium	6
Ready-To-Eat Breakfast Cereals, Fortified		
Product 19, Total	1 ounce each	60
King Vitaman	1 ounce	36
Corn flakes, Rice Chex, Wheaties	1 ounce each	15

Vitamin C (Ascorbic Acid)

VITAMIN C CONTENT OF COMMON FOODS*

Food	Quantity	Milligrams of Vitamin C
Beverages		
Hawaiian Punch-Cherry	6 ounces	60
Hi-C (various flavors)	6 ounces	60
Ocean Spray Cranberry Juice Cocktail	6 ounces	60
Tang (dissolved per directions)	4 ounces	60
Welch's Grape Juice	6 ounces	60
Super Mott's Prune Juice	6 ounces	42
Hawaiian Punch-Very Berry, Fruit Juicy Red	6 ounces	30
Welchade Grape Drink	6 ounces	27

*Milk and milk products, cereal foods (unless fortified), and meats contain little or no ascorbic acid. Organ meats are exceptions. Beef liver contains 23 mg ascorbic acid in a three-ounce serving.

Compiled from: product labels and U.S.D.A. *Home and Garden Bulletin No. 72,* Washington, D.C., revised April, 1977.

Vitamin C (Ascorbic Acid)

GOOD SOURCES OF VITAMIN C

This table lists a variety of foods that are good sources of vitamin C. The best sources of vitamin C are fruits — especially citrus fruits — and vegetables. Milk and milk products provide little vitamin C. Meats, other than organ meats (liver and kidney), have no vitamin C; nor do cereal products unless fortified. The U.S. RDA for adults and children over four for vitamin C is 60 mg.

Food	Quantity	Percent of U.S. RDA
Currants; black, European, raw	1 cup	550.00
Strawberries, frozen	1 carton (10 ounces)	250.00
Brussels sprouts, cooked	1 cup	225.00
Orange juice, fresh	1 cup	206.67
Orange juice; frozen concentrate, diluted	1 cup	200.00
Lemon juice, fresh	1 cup	186.67
Orange-grapefruit juice; frozen concentrate, diluted	1 cup	170.00
Papayas, raw	1 cup (½-inch cubes)	170.00
Orange juice; canned, unsweetened	1 cup	166.67
Grapefruit juice; frozen concentrate, unsweetened, diluted	1 cup	160.00
Green peppers; sweet, raw (without stem or seeds)	1 pod (⅕ pound)	156.67
Grapefruit juice, fresh	1 cup	153.33
Cantaloupe	½ medium	150.00
Honeydew melon	½ medium	148.33
Strawberries, raw	1 cup	146.67
Collards, cooked	1 cup	145.00
Grapefruit juice; canned, white, unsweetened	1 cup	140.00

Vitamin C (Ascorbic Acid)

GOOD SOURCES OF VITAMIN C

Food	Quantity	Percent of U.S. RDA
Lime juice, fresh	1 cup	131.67
Grapefruit, canned in syrup	1 cup	126.67
Broccoli, cooked	½ cup	116.67
Peppers; sweet, boiled, drained	1 pod	116.67
Cress; garden, raw	3½ ounces	115.00
Kale, cooked (leaves and stems)	1 cup	113.33
Mustard greens, cooked	1 cup	113.33
Turnip greens, cooked	1 cup	113.33
Cauliflower, cooked (flowerbuds)	1 cup	110.00
Oranges, raw (all varieties)	1 orange (2 ⅝" diameter)	110.00
Dandelion greens, raw	1 cup	105.00
Raspberries; red, frozen	1 carton (10 ounces)	98.33
Tangerine juice; canned, sweetened	1 cup	91.67
Lime juice; canned, unsweetened	1 cup	86.67
Casaba melon	½ medium	83.33
Spinach, cooked	1 cup	83.33
Cabbage, cooked (common varieties)	1 cup	80.00
Grapefruit; raw, pink or red	½ medium	73.33
Grapefruit; raw, white	½ medium	73.33
Avocado, raw (late summer, fall: Florida)	1 whole	71.67
Cabbage; red, raw	1 cup	71.67
Cabbage, raw (common variety)	1 cup	70.00
Kale; boiled, drained	1 cup	70.00
Tomatoes, raw	1 tomato (3-inch diameter)	70.00

Vitamin C (Ascorbic Acid)

GOOD SOURCES OF VITAMIN C

Food	Quantity	Percent of U.S. RDA
Tomatoes, canned (solids and liquid)	1 cup	68.33
Cranberry juice cocktail, canned	1 cup	66.67
Orange-apricot juice drink	1 cup	66.67
Potato sticks	3½ ounces	66.67
Cabbage; savoy, raw	1 cup	65.00
Lemon, raw	1 lemon (2 ⅛-inch diameter)	65.00
Tomato juice, canned	1 cup	65.00
Asparagus; green, canned (solids and liquid)	1 cup	61.67
Elderberries, raw	3½ ounces	60.00
Strawberry pie	1 sector	56.67
Turnips; cooked, diced	1 cup	56.67
Peas; green, cooked	1 cup	55.00
Sauerkraut, canned (solids and liquid)	1 cup	55.00
Dandelion greens, cooked	1 cup	53.33
Raspberries; red, raw	1 cup	51.67
Avocado, raw (mid-late winter: California)	1 whole	50.00
Blackberries, raw	1 cup	50.00
Sweet potatoes, canned	1 cup	50.00
Watermelon, raw	1 wedge (4 by 8 inches)	50.00
Beans; lima, cooked, drained	1 cup	48.33
Cole slaw with French dressing (commercial)	3½ ounces	48.33
French dressing (homemade)	3½ ounces	48.33
Lettuce; raw, iceberg	1 head (4¾-inch diameter)	48.33

Vitamin C (Ascorbic Acid)

GOOD SOURCES OF VITAMIN C

Food	Quantity	Percent of U.S. RDA
Mayonnaise	3½ ounces	48.33
Cowpeas, cooked	1 cup	46.67
Peaches; dried, uncooked	1 cup	46.67
Tangerines, raw	1 medium	45.00
Winter squash; baked, mashed	1 cup	45.00
Cabbage; spoon or bok choy, cooked	1 cup	43.33
Sweet potatoes, boiled (peeled after boiling)	1 medium	41.67
Cherries; sweet, raw	1 cup	40.00
Pineapple; raw, diced	1 cup	40.00
Spinach, canned (drained solids)	1 cup	40.00
Sweet potatoes, baked (peeled after baking)	1 medium	40.00
Beef liver, fried	3 ounces	38.33
Cucumbers; raw, pared	1 cucumber (10 ounces)	38.33
Beet greens; cooked, drained (leaves and stems)	1 cup	36.67
Peas; green, canned (solids and liquid)	1 cup	36.67
Pineapple juice, canned	1 cup	36.67
Spaghetti with meat balls, tomato sauce (homemade)	1 cup	36.67
Summer squash; cooked, diced	1 cup	35.00
Blueberries, raw	1 cup	33.33
Potatoes, baked (peeled after baking)	1 medium	33.33
Potatoes, boiled (peeled before boiling)	1 medium	33.33
Apricot halves; dried, uncooked	1 cup	31.67
Cabbage; celery or Chinese, raw	1 cup	31.67

Vitamin C (Ascorbic Acid)

GOOD SOURCES OF VITAMIN C

Food	Quantity	Percent of U.S. RDA
Potatoes, mashed (milk added)	1 cup	31.67
Lettuce; Boston, raw	1 head (4-inch diameter)	30.00
Lettuce, cos or romaine	3½ ounces	30.00
Potatoes, mashed (milk and butter added)	1 cup	30.00
Tomato-vegetable soup with noodles, dehydrated	1 package (2½-ounces)	30.00
Leeks, raw (bulb and lower leaf)	3½ ounces	28.33
Lemonade concentrate, diluted	1 cup	28.33
Okra, cooked	8 pods	28.33
Rhubarb, cooked (sugar added)	1 cup	28.33
Soybeans; boiled, drained	3½ ounces	28.33
Sweet potatoes, candied	1 potato	28.33
Asparagus; cooked, drained	4 spears	26.67
Parsnips, cooked	1 cup	26.67
Beans; snap, green; cooked, drained	1 cup	25.00
Beef and vegetable stew	1 cup	25.00
Lobster salad	3 ounces	25.00
Spanish rice (homemade)	3½ ounces	25.00
Tomato soup; canned, condensed (with equal amount milk)	1 cup	25.00

Compiled from CONSUMER GUIDE® magazine Nutrition Data Bank.

Vitamin A (Retinol)

As far as vitamin A is concerned, the eyes have it. The essential nutrient known as vitamin A (retinol) plays a vital role in vision, especially in the ability to see in dim light, and to keep the outer layers of the eye healthy. Without it, people have trouble seeing at night, and the eyes may become dry and cloudy.

History

As indicated by its position at the head of the "vitamin alphabet," vitamin A was the first to be "found". It was discovered in the early 1900s after researchers recognized that a certain substance in animal fats and fish oils was necessary for the growth of young animals. Because it was found in animal fats, the substance was originally called "fat-soluble A." Its name was soon changed to vitamin A.

Vitamin A includes several compounds that have similar biological activity: retinol and the carotenes. Retinol is

Vitamin A (Retinol)

vitamin A as we know it; it is the natural form of the vitamin that is found in animal foods. Carotenes are provitamins, substances the body can use to manufacture a vitamin. They occur in plant foods.

Food Sources of Vitamin A

Liver is the best single food source of vitamin A, but whole milk, fortified skim milk, butter, and margarine are good sources. Red palm oil, used in cooking in many tropical countries, and fish liver oils are rich in vitamin A.

Orange and yellow fruits and vegetables have high vitamin A values because of the carotenes present. Generally, the darker the vegetable, the more the carotene. Carrots, for example, are particularly good sources of carotene and, therefore, they have high vitamin A "value." Green, leafy vegetables have high carotene contents, but the yellow-orange pigment is masked by the green chlorophyll. According to the Food and Nutrition Board, the usual American mixed diet contains about half the vitamin A (as retinol) in animal foods and half (as carotenes) in plant foods. (See the first and second tables at the end of this chapter for the vitamin A content of some common foods and for a list of good food sources of vitamin A and the percent of the U.S. RDA they provide.

Dietary Requirements for Vitamin A

The Recommended Dietary Allowance (RDA) for vitamin A is 5,000 international units (IU) for men and 4,000 IU for women. The RDAs for children range from 2,000 to 3,500 IU. While they are growing rapidly, children are susceptible to vitamin A deficiency and the eye problems it may cause.

You don't need to follow the RDAs to the letter each day. But you must be sure to get adequate quantities of the vitamin in the long run. For example, if you eat liver or carrots on one day, your intake of vitamin A is much higher than the RDA, and you can make up for not meeting the

Vitamin A (Retinol)

RDA the day before. If most of the vitamin A in your diet comes from retinol in animal foods, you can get by with less than the RDA, but if you're a vegetarian and get all the vitamin A from carotenes in vegetables, you should exceed the RDA.

Finally, because vitamin A is not soluble in water, excess amounts of the vitamin do not leave the body in the urine but accumulate in the liver. This storehouse of vitamin A can be tapped whenever the dietary intake of the vitamin falls too low. For most adults it would take months without vitamin A in the diet to deplete this storehouse.

You don't have to follow the RDA for vitamin A rigidly, but you still need adequate amounts of it. With a balanced diet that includes milk, butter or margarine, and yellow or green vegetables, you should have no trouble. (The third table at the end of this chapter shows the vitamin A content in two typical daily diets.)

Function of Vitamin A

Vitamin A's role in vision involves a biochemical reaction within the cells of the eye's retina. When vitamin A is oxidized, one of its products combines with proteins to form compounds, photoreceptors, in the cells. Photoreceptors in the eye's retina pick up visual signals in both bright and dim light and transform them into electrical impulses which are transmitted to the brain. Although photoreceptors for both day and night vision make use of vitamin A, the cells that work in dim light are especially vulnerable to any deficiency. These cells, the cell rods, rapidly use up vitamin A. If the vitamin is not replaced, night blindness results.

Apart from its effect on vision, vitamin A also helps maintain the physical soundness of the eye itself. With a vitamin A deficiency, the outer part of the eye—the tough, transparent coating called the cornea, and the "whites" of the eyes, or conjunctiva—become dry, a condition called xerophthalmia. If it continues unchecked, irreversible

Vitamin A (Retinol)

damage and blindness may follow.

Vitamin A is necessary for normal growth and reproduction. The vitamin is required to maintain the health of the skin and of the linings of the gastrointestinal and respiratory tracts.

Deficiency of Vitamin A

Night blindness, the inability to see well in dim light, is the first symptom of vitamin A deficiency. Later, the outer layers of the eyes become dry, thickened, and cloudy. Severe vitamin A deficiency causes blindness.

The skin becomes dry and rough, developing a "goose flesh" appearance. Vitamin A deficiency increases susceptibility to infectious diseases because the linings of the gastrointestinal and respiratory tracts are damaged and can't act as barriers to keep bacteria from entering the body.

To prevent the consequences of deficiency, some developing countries have introduced programs to encourage people to eat foods with a high vitamin A value. In many countries, for example, liver and dairy products are scarce or expensive, so people are taught to select plant foods with carotenes and to eat plenty of them. Some countries are beginning to fortify foods; vitamin A-fortified sugar has been introduced in some Central American countries. Others provide large doses of the vitamin (200,000 IU) to children at six-month intervals.

Therapeutic Uses of Vitamin A

Physicians prescribe large initial doses of vitamin A (100,000 IU) to treat children with xerophthalmia. Since the condition can rapidly become very serious, physicians administer large doses for the first few days but then reduce them. Usually after three days, the dosage is decreased to 25,000 to 50,000 IU.

Vitamin A (Retinol)

Diseases such as obstructive jaundice or cystic fibrosis cause poor absorption of dietary fat and fat-soluble vitamins. People who have such diseases may take adequate amounts of vitamin A in their diets but still develop a deficiency because the disease hampers the absorption of the vitamin into the body. For such patients, physicians often prescribe vitamin A supplements providing 5 to 10 times the RDA to overcome or prevent vitamin A deficiency.

A disease that is accompanied by prolonged fever—infectious hepatitis or rheumatic fever, for example—may rapidly deplete the liver's reserves of vitamin A. Sometimes, as part of the treatment of these diseases, physicians prescribe vitamin A in excess of the RDA so deficiency will not occur.

Hazards and Toxicity of Vitamin A

With vitamin A, one massive dose or large doses over an extended period of time can cause loss of appetite and hair, headaches, blurred vision, and dry, flaky skin. They even may cause hemorrhaging. This is true for retinol, derivatives of which are used in vitamin supplements. Carotenes are not toxic.

Estimates of the amount of vitamin A that will cause toxicity vary. But toxic reactions have followed single doses of two million international units in adults and 75,000 IU in children. And continued use of doses 5 to 10 times the RDA is risky.[1]

The danger of toxicity may be compounded by overage, manufacturers' practice of including in supplements more than the labeled amount of some vitamins to ensure the vitamins' stated potency throughout its shelf-life. For example, the overage may be as high as 40 percent for vitamin A; that is, a supplement with a labeled dose of 25,000 IU may provide as much as 35,000 IU.[2] These additional amounts increase the risk of overdose.

Vitamin A (Retinol)

Claims and Controversy

Fortunately, claims for using supplemental vitamin A are not widespread. But the fact that supplements containing 25,000 IU per capsule are readily available to the consumer seems to imply that large amounts of the vitamin might be useful. The individual unaware of the hazards of toxicity might be tempted to take several of these each day with the hope of benefit.

Nutrition author Adelle Davis recommended supplements of at least 25,000 IU daily, pointing out that amounts over 50,000 IU daily could be toxic.[3] But then she added that the damage could be prevented or corrected by an increased vitamin C intake. She did not specify how much of an increase. We know of no data to support this claim.

Davis also stated, "Tests have shown that persons having auto accidents at night are pathologically deficient in this vitamin." This served to dramatize the results of inadequate intakes of the vitamin. A person with night blindness would have difficulty in driving at night, but we know of no data even suggesting that nighttime automobile accidents are mainly the result of vitamin A deficiency.

Vitamin A supplements with large doses of the vitamin have been used to treat acne. The Food and Drug Administration's Advisory Panel on Vitamin and Mineral Drug Products for Over-the-Counter Human Use concluded that clinical tests failed to prove that vitamin A was useful for treating acne.[2] The panel further concluded that vitamin A supplements are of no value in treating dry or wrinkled skin, respiratory diseases, or visual defects and diseases of the eye, since these conditions are generally not related to a deficiency of the vitamin.

CONSUMER GUIDE® magazine Opinion

We wish to emphasize that large doses of vitamin A can be toxic. So don't take chances with massive doses of the vitamin in supplement form. You can easily get all the

Vitamin A (Retinol)

vitamin A you need by eating a variety of foods and including yellow-orange or dark green vegetables several times a week. While toxicity from single massive doses of vitamin A is a rare occurrence, there is good documentation of toxicity from long use of large amounts of the vitamin.

Vitamin A Summary

Type of vitamin: Fat-soluble
Where stored in the body: Liver
Length of storage: Long-term (months)
History: First vitamin discovered (1912)
Food sources: Liver is the best food source. Yellow-orange fruits and vegetables and dark green, leafy vegetables, whole milk, vitamin A-fortified skim milk, butter, and margarine are good sources.
Recommended Dietary Allowance: Women: 4,000 IU; men: 5,000 IU
Function: Necessary to see in dim light, for normal growth and reproduction, and to maintain health of the skin, the linings of the gastrointestinal and respiratory tracts, and the outer layers of the eye
Deficiency: Results in night blindness; dryness of the outer layers of the eye (xerophthalmia), which may lead to blindness; dry, rough skin; reduced resistance to infectious diseases
Hazards and toxicity: Supplements containing large doses of vitamin A can cause loss of appetite, headache, blurred vision, loss of hair, and dry, flaky skin.
Claims and controversy: There is no evidence that amounts of vitamin A in excess of the RDAs are needed or are of any benefit in treating diseases or conditions not caused by a deficiency of the vitamin.
CONSUMER GUIDE® magazine opinion: Supplements of vitamin A should be used to prevent or treat deficiency when need is determined by a physician. Large doses of the vitamin can be toxic. Don't take chances.

Vitamin A (Retinol)

VITAMIN A CONTENT OF COMMON FOODS

Food	Quantity	IU of Vitamin A
Milk Group		
Ice cream	1 cup	540
Milk, skim (fortified with vitamin A)	8 ounces	500
Cottage cheese	1 cup	350
Milk, whole	8 ounces	310
Cheddar cheese	1 ounce	300
Yogurt, whole milk	1 cup	280
Cheese, processed, American	1 ounce	260
Swiss cheese	1 ounce	240
Ice milk	1 cup	210
Yogurt, skim milk	1 cup	20
Fats and Oils		
Margarine (fortified)	1 tablespoon	470
Butter	1 tablespoon	430
Meat Group		
Beef liver	3 ounces	45,380
Egg	1 whole	260
(Other meats have little or no vitamin A)		
Cereal Group		
Ready-to-eat breakfast cereals (fortified)		
Total, Product 19	1 ounce each	5,000
King Vitaman	1 ounce	2,500
Wheaties, corn flakes, Grape Nuts Flakes, raisin bran	1 ounce each	1,250
Fruits		
Cantaloupe, fresh	½ melon	9,240

Vitamin A (Retinol)

VITAMIN A CONTENT OF COMMON FOODS

Food	Quantity	IU of Vitamin A
Apricots, canned	1 cup	4,490
Peach	1 medium	1,330
Banana	1 medium	230
Apple	1 medium	120
Strawberries, fresh	1 cup	90
Vegetables		
Sweet potato, baked	1 medium	9,230
Carrot, raw	1 medium	7,930
Squash; winter, mashed	½ cup	4,300
Tomato, fresh	1 medium	2,170
Broccoli, cooked	½ cup	2,000
Asparagus, cooked	½ cup	700
Green or snap beans, cooked	½ cup	350
Corn; sweet, frozen, cooked	½ cup	290

Compiled from: product labels and U.S.D.A. *Home and Garden Bulletin No. 72,* Washington, D.C., revised April, 1977.

Vitamin A (Retinol)

GOOD SOURCES OF VITAMIN A

This table lists a variety of food that are good sources of vitamin A. Liver is the best single food source of vitamin A. Whole milk, fortified skim milk, butter, and margarine are good sources. Orange and yellow fruits and vegetables and green, leafy vegetables are also good sources. The U.S. RDA for adults and children over four for vitamin A is 5,000 IU.

Food	Quantity	Percent of U.S. RDA
Beef liver, fried	2 ounces	605.60
Dandelion greens, raw	1 cup	504.00
Dandelion greens, cooked	1 cup	421.20
Sweet potatoes, canned	1 cup	340.00
Apricot halves; dried, uncooked	1 cup	327.00
Pumpkin, canned	1 cup	291.80
Spinach, cooked	1 cup	291.60
Spinach; canned, drained	1 cup	288.00
Sweet potatoes, boiled (peeled after boiling)	1 medium	232.20
Sweet potatoes, candied	1 potato	220.60
Collards, cooked	1 cup	205.20
Red hot peppers, dried (without seeds)	1 tablespoon	195.00
Cress; garden, raw	3½ ounces	186.00
Peas and carrots, frozen (boiled, drained)	3½ ounces	186.00
Kale; boiled, drained	1 cup	180.40
Sweet potatos, baked (peeled after baking)	1 medium	178.20
Winter squash, baked (mashed)	1 cup	172.20
Apricots; dried, cooked, unsweetened (fruit and liquid)	1 cup	171.00
Turnip greens, cooked	1 cup	165.40

Vitamin A (Retinol)

GOOD SOURCES OF VITAMIN A

Food	Quantity	Percent of U.S. RDA
Kale, cooked (leaves and stems)	1 cup	162.80
Mustard greens, cooked	1 cup	162.40
Beet greens; cooked, drained (leaves and stems)	1 cup	148.00
Cantaloupe	½ medium	130.80
Peaches; dried, uncooked	1 cup	124.80
Carrot, raw	1 whole	110.00
Cabbage; spoon or bok choy, cooked	1 cup	105.40
Apricots, canned in heavy syrup	1 cup	90.20
Broccoli; cooked, drained	1 medium stalk	90.00
Butter	½ cup	75.00
Margarine	½ cup	75.00
Peach halves; dried, cooked, unsweetened (fruit and liquid)	1 cup	65.80
Papayas, raw	1 cup (½-inch cubes)	63.80
Sweet potato pie	1 sector	62.40
Chicken pot pie, baked	1 pie (pre-bake weight, 8 ounces)	60.40
Plums, canned with syrup	1 cup	59.40
Vegetarian soups; canned, condensed (with equal amount water)	1 cup	58.80
Apricots, raw	3 apricots	57.80
Vegetable beef soup; canned, condensed (with equal amount water)	1 cup	54.00
Watermelon, raw	1 wedge (4 by 8 inches)	50.20
Minestrone soup; canned, condensed (with equal amount water)	1 cup	47.00

Vitamin A (Retinol)

GOOD SOURCES OF VITAMIN A

Food	Quantity	Percent of U.S. RDA
Beef and vegetable stew	1 cup	46.20
Tomatoes, canned (solids and liquid)	1 cup	43.40
Tomato juice, canned	1 cup	38.80
Sour cream	1 cup	38.60
Lettuce, cos or romaine	3½ ounces	38.00
Endive, curly (including escarole)	2 ounces	37.40
Beef pot pie, baked	1 pie (pre-bake weight, 8 ounces)	37.20
Prunes; dried, medium, cooked, unsweetened	1 cup	37.20
Crab, steamed	3 ounces	36.90
Palm oil	1 tablespoon	36.62
Swordfish, broiled with butter or oleo	3 ounces	35.00
Lake whitefish; stuffed, baked	3 ounces	34.00
Tomato-vegetable soup with noodles, dehydrated	1 package (2½ ounces)	34.00
Cherries; red, sour, pitted (canned with water)	1 cup	33.20
Tomatoes, raw	1 medium	32.80
Spaghetti with meat balls, tomato sauce (homemade)	1 cup	31.80
Orange-apricot juice drink	1 cup	28.80
Finnan haddie	3 ounces	27.38
Peaches, raw	1 medium	26.40
Liverwurst, fresh	2 slices (¼-inch thick)	25.40
Milk, skim (fortified with vitamin A)	1 cup	10.00
Milk, whole	1 cup	6.20

Compiled from: CONSUMER GUIDE® magazine Nutrition Data Bank.

Vitamin A (Retinol)

VITAMIN A CONTENT IN TWO DAILY DIETS

Typical Day's Diet for Woman (1,700 Calories)	IU of Vitamin A
Breakfast	
4 ounces orange juice	270
1 ounce enriched corn flakes	1,250
1 slice enriched white toast	none
1 pat butter	150
1 cup 2-percent milk	500
Black coffee	none
Lunch	
Sandwich: 2 slices whole-wheat bread, 1 slice American cheese, 2 ounces boiled ham	490
1 cup skim milk (fortified)	500
½ cup cole slaw	60
Dinner	
½ chicken breast, fried	70
1 medium baked potato	none
1 cup tossed green salad	180
½ cup peas, cooked	480
1 enriched dinner roll	none
2 pats butter	300
½ cup ice cream	270
Black coffee	none
Total	**4,520**
RDA	**4,000**

Compiled from: U.S.D.A. *Home and Garden Bulletin No. 72*, Washington, D.C., revised April, 1977.

Vitamin A (Retinol)

VITAMIN A CONTENT IN TWO DAILY DIETS

Typical Day's Diet for Teenage Boy (3,000 Calories)	IU of Vitamin A
Breakfast	
½ medium pink grapefruit	540
2 scrambled eggs	620
2 slices enriched white toast	none
1 pat butter	150
1 cup whole milk	310
Lunch	
1 cheeseburger	360
2 cups whole milk	620
10 large French-fried potatoes	none
1 medium banana	230
Dinner	
4 ounces round steak	25
1 cup green beans	780
1 cup mashed potatoes	40
Lettuce and tomato salad	400
2 slices enriched white bread	none
1 pat butter	150
1 cup whole milk	310
4 chocolate chip cookies	50
Snacks	
Cola drink	none
½ cup ice cream	270
¼ of 14-inch cheese pizza	200
Total	**5,055**
RDA	**5,000**

Compiled from: U.S.D.A. *Home and Garden Bulletin No. 72*, Washington, D.C., revised April, 1977.

Vitamin D

Fifty years ago, few children in tropical countries developed malformed bones and teeth from rickets, but many in temperate climates and large industrial cities did. The reason for the difference was sunshine and sunshine vitamin D.

The children in tropical countries were exposed to sunlight year-round, and their skin could form the substance that was needed to prevent poor bone and tooth development—vitamin D. Children in temperate zones got little exposure to the sun during the winter months, and their skin could not make enough vitamin D. Neither could the skin of children in large, industrial cities, because the smoke-filled air filtered out much of the sun's ultraviolet light.

Vitamin D

Nowadays, the malformed bones and teeth that are symptoms of the disease known as rickets are seldom seen in the United States. The incidence of rickets has been cut dramatically by the increased availability of milk fortified with vitamin D. Milk was chosen as the medium for vitamin D in this country because children usually drink it in quantity. Milk also was selected because it is the single best source of calcium in the American diet—what better place to add the vitamin necessary for the utilization of calcium? Proof of the effectiveness of the vitamin D-fortification program is the virtual disappearance of rickets in the United States. Today when rickets is found, it usually can be traced to poverty, neglect, or ignorance.

History

Rickets afflicted large numbers of children in this country in the early 1900s. While searching for the cause of the disease, researchers fed various diets to experimental animals. Some of the diets prevented calcium from depositing in the bones and produced the characteristic soft bones of rickets. From this research, investigators concluded that rickets actually was a vitamin deficiency. But they became perplexed when they discovered that ultraviolet light also played a part. Nutritionists in the 1920s found that rickets could be prevented or cured by feeding children cod liver oil or food that had been exposed to ultraviolet light, and could be prevented by exposing children to direct sunlight or the light from a sunlamp. The explanation for these findings did not come for several years.

Cod liver oil was effective in the treatment of rickets because it contained vitamin D. Ultraviolet light changed a substance in plant foods, ergosterol, into a form of the vitamin called vitamin D_2. Therefore, ultraviolet light provided the essential nutrient in plant foods where none existed before. Direct sunlight and ultraviolet light from a sunlamp also provided vitamin D by transforming a

Vitamin D

substance found in the human skin into vitamin D_3. The vitamin D_3 from the skin then traveled to other parts of the body.

Food Sources and Dietary Requirements for Vitamin D

Children who are unable to make enough vitamin D because the climate or environmental conditions reduce their exposure to the sun need a dietary source of vitamin D during the period of growth and development. No naturally occurring foods other than some fish and fish liver oils contain significant amounts of the vitamin. To provide this essential nutrient for children, foods have been fortified with vitamin D. Today, many ready-to-eat breakfast cereals contain about 40 international units (IU) of vitamin D in a one-ounce serving. Essentially, all the evaporated (when diluted), whole, and skim milk sold in this country has 10 times that much vitamin D in each quart. Skim milk powder mixed with water provides the same amount of the vitamin as does whole milk. The amount of vitamin D in a quart of milk—whether evaporated (diluted), whole, or skim—coincides with the Food and Nutrition Board's Recommended Dietary Allowance (RDA) of 400 IU for those under age 22.

According to the Food and Nutrition Board, before bone development is complete, children, teens, and young adults should receive 400 IU of vitamin D each day. Because of the definite need for the vitamin during growth, mothers are encouraged to provide their infants and children with vitamin D in an amount approximating 400 IU daily.

When bone development is complete the daily requirement for vitamin D can be met by exposure to sunlight (No RDA has been established for adults other than for pregnant or lactating women.) Those who are seldom exposed to sunshine by reason of occupation, living habits, or mode of dress probably should drink vitamin D-fortified milk regularly to ensure an adequate intake.

Vitamin D

Function of Vitamin D

Vitamin D is necessary for the body to absorb and use calcium, a major component of bones and teeth. Without vitamin D, calcium cannot be absorbed into the body.

Vitamin D in the body, absorbed from food or made in the skin, first travels to the liver, where it undergoes a chemical change. In its new form vitamin D moves through the bloodstream to the kidney, where it undergoes another change. This second-generation vitamin D derivative is carried to the cells lining the intestine and directs them to produce calcium-binding protein. True to its name, the calcium-binding protein attaches to the calcium and carries it past obstructive cell membranes and into the body. This protein facilitates the absorption of calcium.

Deficiency of Vitamin D

Rickets, or vitamin D deficiency in children, is responsible for poor development of bones and teeth. One of its most common signs is bowlegs, which occur when leg bones become so weak that they cannot support a child's weight and bend outward as the child begins to walk. Another common sign is bead-like swellings on the ribs, a condition known as rachitic rosary. Also, teething is late, and teeth are susceptible to decay. If the disease is treated promptly, some bone abnormalities can be corrected.

Osteomalacia, or vitamin D deficiency in adults, is responsible for the loss of calcium from the bones, which become weak and susceptible to fracture. Osteomalacia occurs most frequently among women in developing countries who have had several pregnancies followed by long periods of nursing, and who have low calcium and vitamin D intakes.

Therapeutic Uses of Vitamin D

Supplemental vitamin D, in a dose of 3,000 to 5,000 IU a

Vitamin D

day, is a physician's standard treatment of rickets and osteomalacia. A dose of 50,000 IU of vitamin D plus calcium supplements may be used by physicians to treat osteomalacia complicated by intestinal disorders causing poor absorption. For both diseases, vitamin D is accompanied by an increased milk intake of one to two pints per day. The FDA Advisory Panel on Vitamin and Mineral Drug Products for Over-the-Counter Human Use concluded that supplements containing 400 IU of vitamin D are suitable to prevent a deficiency; higher dosage supplements should be available only by prescription.[1]

Physicians have used large doses of the vitamin with some success to treat patients with genetic disorders that cause defective calcium or phosphorus metabolism. And they have managed some of these diseases with small doses of the derivatives of vitamin D; that is, compounds similar to those produced in the body by the liver and the kidney.

Treatment with derivatives of the vitamin has been effective also in normalizing calcium metabolism for patients with severe kidney disease, who often absorb calcium poorly and have low blood levels of the mineral.

Hazards and Toxicity of Vitamin D

Too much vitamin D can be toxic. Large doses of the vitamin cause large amounts of calcium to be absorbed. The mineral accumulates in body tissues, sometimes causing irreversible damage to the kidneys. Therefore, physicians should not administer massive doses of the vitamin unless the amount of calcium in the patient's blood is measured frequently. If the amount of calcium in the blood becomes too high, the vitamin treatment should be stopped to allow the level to return to normal.

Prolonged intake of 2,000 IU of vitamin D (five times the RDA) can cause dangerously high blood levels of calcium in infants and children. Such high intakes probably cannot be obtained from food alone, but overzealous use of cod

Vitamin D

liver oil or vitamin D supplements, plus vitamin D-fortified milk and foods, could conceivably push the daily intake up to 2,000 IU.

Some years ago in this country, nutritionists were concerned about the very real danger of vitamin D toxicity.[2] Vitamin supplements for infants in the early 1960s contained as much as 1,000 IU in a daily dose. Furthermore, many infant foods were fortified with the vitamin. For example, chocolate flavorings for milk were fortified with enough vitamin D to furnish 100 to 150 IU per glass, and many breakfast cereals contained as much as 400 IU in one serving. By using a supplement with 1,000 IU and fortified foods (plus fortified milk), some children theoretically could have got as much as 4,700 IU per day. Fearful of the consequences of high intakes of the vitamin, nutritionists urged manufacturers to reduce the amount of vitamin D in vitamin supplements and foods commonly eaten by children. The manufacturers agreed and a potential problem was averted.

Today, there is still some concern about vitamin D toxicity. Some vitamin supplements available in health food stores contain 1,000 IU of vitamin D in a daily dose. Examples are the Natural Sales Company's Vitamin D Capsules and Super Vitamin A and D Capsules, and Essential Organics' Omniplex and Ultraplex. Companies that produce supplements often add more than the labeled amount of the vitamin so the supplement will not contain less than its labeled amount during its shelf-life. These supplements may furnish 1,500 to 2,000 IU in a daily dose at the time of manufacture.[2]

The risk of adverse effects or toxicity from overuse of vitamin D supplements containing such high doses is real.

Claims and Controversy

Catharyn Elwood, in *Feel Like a Million*, states that large doses of vitamin D have been reported as successful against arthritis and that a deficiency of vitamin D can

Vitamin D

cause tension responsible for myopia (near-sightedness). She included vitamin D among the nutrients necessary for nerve stability and recommended that a person never take less than one hour of sunbathing or 800 to 4,000 IU of vitamin D daily.[3]

Although she commented on the known toxicity of vitamin D, Adelle Davis recommended that children be given daily doses of cod liver oil in amounts which would provide much more than the RDA of vitamin D.[4] Practicing what she preached, Davis took 5,000 IU of the vitamin daily. She claimed that natural vitamin D, such as that present in cod liver oil, is not toxic.

The authors of *Psychodietetics* suggest that a good multivitamin supplement should contain from 1,000 to 2,500 IU per daily dose.[5] They further note: "The few studies to date which seem to support a vitamin A and vitamin D toxicity potential used fantastically large quantities to demonstrate an ill effect. You'd have to sit down and plan your own demise to take a damaging dose of these nutrients."

We believe that the high doses recommended by these writers could, over a period of time, be hazardous and could cause problems such as those described in the section on toxicity. The lack of toxicity attributed to natural vitamin D is contradicted by documented cases of hypervitaminosis D in children who were given large amounts of cod liver oil. There is no evidence supporting the use of vitamin D for treatment of any condition not related to deficiency of the vitamin.

CONSUMER GUIDE® magazine Opinion

We concur with the Food and Nutrition Board which emphasizes that there is no known benefit from vitamin D in excess of the RDA, but there is known hazard.[6] Supplements that contain vitamin D in excess of 400 IU should be avoided. Children and adolescents, who particu-

Vitamin D

larly need vitamin D and calcium for proper growth, should drink three to four glasses of vitamin D-fortified milk daily.

Vitamin D Summary

Type of vitamin: Fat-soluble
Where stored in the body: In liver and, to some extent, other tissues.
History: Discovered in the 1930s
Food sources: Unless fortified, no food except some fish and fish liver oils contains significant amounts of the vitamin. Vitamin D-fortified milk is principal source in American diet.
Recommended Dietary Allowance: 400 IU for those under age 22 and for pregnant women and nursing mothers; no RDA for people over age 22
Function: Essential for absorption of calcium
Deficiency: Results in poor bone and tooth development in children (rickets); loss of calcium from bones in adults (osteomalacia).
Therapeutic uses: Physicians prescribe vitamin D supplements to treat rickets and osteomalacia. Genetic disorders characterized by defective calcium and/or phosphorus metabolism and severe kidney disease are treated with vitamin D and its metabolic derivatives.
Hazards and toxicity: Excess amounts of vitamin D cause absorption of abnormally large amounts of calcium, which become deposited in body tissues. Irreversible damage to the kidney may result.
Claims and controversy: Claims that vitamin D is effective against arthritis and nervousness are unfounded.
CONSUMER GUIDE® magazine opinion: There is no known benefit from excess amounts of vitamin D. But there is known hazard. We advise that you not take supplements containing in excess of 400 IU. Better still, children and adolescents should drink three to four glasses of fortified milk a day to reach the RDA.

Vitamin E (Tocopherol)

If ever a vitamin has received more credit than it deserves, vitamin E is it. Retail sales of vitamin E have soared and continue to increase even though there is no scientific evidence that daily doses over the Recommended Dietary Allowance (RDA) promote physical endurance, enhance sexual potency, prevent heart attacks, slow the aging process, or produce any of the other minor miracles attributed to it. Millions of consumers, despite scientific information to the contrary, remain devoted to vitamin E and refuse to replace faith and the fiction of false publicity with fact.

Vitamin E (Tocopherol)

What exactly is vitamin E? What can it do? And how did it gain its reputation as a miracle worker?

History

The first indication for the existence of vitamin E came in 1922. Laboratory rats fed purified diets lost their reproductive ability; male rats became sterile and female rats reabsorbed their fetuses or were delivered of deformed or stillborn offspring. When foods such as lettuce, wheat, meat, or butter were added to the animals' diets, an unknown factor was supplied which prevented these reproductive problems. Isolated in 1936, the factor was named "tocopherol" from the Greek, meaning, "to bring forth offspring." Later the substance became known as vitamin E.

It was discovered that vitamin E is not a single compound. There are several different compounds, all with vitamin E activity. One, known as alpha-tocopherol, has the greatest activity. (Its derivative, alpha-tocopherol acetate, is commonly used in commercial supplements.) Other compounds with vitamin E activity are beta-tocopherol, gamma-tocopherol and delta-tocopherol.

Following the discovery of vitamin E, deficiency studies were conducted using various animal species. It soon became obvious that deficiency symptoms varied from one species to another. In rabbits a degenerative muscle disease was the result of vitamin E deficiency, and the symptoms were corrected by the addition of the vitamin to the animals' diets. Because these symptoms were similar to those seen in human subjects with muscular dystrophy, researchers hoped that that crippling disease in humans could be cured or prevented with vitamin E. It was hoped, too, that the vitamin might be helpful in human cases of infertility and sterility. However, studies since 1938 have failed to show any such benefits to people.

Here lies the foundation for the false claims that have surrounded vitamin E as an aid for sexual potency and

Vitamin E (Tocopherol)

muscle disorders. Claims have accumulated over the years.

Food Sources of Vitamin E

Vegetable and seed oils such as those commonly used in cooking and in salad dressings are the best food sources of vitamin E. Corn, cottonseed, soybean, safflower, and wheat germ oils and margarines made from vegetable oils are all good sources of the vitamin. Smaller amounts of vitamin E are present in meats, cereal and dairy products, and vegetables. Whole-grain cereal foods have more vitamin E than refined or processed cereal products, unless the latter are fortified with the vitamin.

Commercial processing of vegetable oils and other foods causes some loss of vitamin E. Also some loss of the vitamin may occur during home storage or cooking of foods. But despite these inevitable losses, a balanced diet supplies vitamin E sufficient to meet people's needs.

Department of Agriculture studies show that the average consumption of vegetable oils and of products made from vegetable oils has steadily increased during the last 30 years. This suggests that people are getting more vitamin E today than they did in the early part of the century.

Several studies have shown, too, that typical diets furnish about 10 to 13 international units (IU) of alpha-tocopherol per day. The total vitamin E value of such diets would be even greater, since vitamin activity is also contributed by other tocopherols.

Dietary Requirements for Vitamin E

Human requirements for vitamin E are difficult to estimate. The determination of the current RDA—12 IU for women and 15 IU for men—is based on information about the average amount of vitamin E activity in usual mixed American diets. People consuming a variety of foods do not exhibit any signs of vitamin E deficiency. Consequent-

Vitamin E (Tocopherol)

ly, it can be assumed they have adequate vitamin E intake.

Vitamin E needs are influenced by the kind and amount of fat in the diet. Both human and animal studies have demonstrated that vitamin E requirements increase when vegetable oils are substituted for animal fats. But since vegetable oils are the best food sources of vitamin E, the new vitamin E needs are met automatically.

Function of Vitamin E

Vitamin E is a fat-soluble vitamin and tends to accumulate in the body, since it is not easily excreted. It is stored to some extent in all body tissues but especially in the fatty tissues.

Vitamin E functions as an antioxidant within the cells and tissues of the body. This means that it helps to prevent undesirable oxidation reactions by inhibiting the combination of a substance with oxygen. For example, it protects the cells from being damaged by products formed when the so-called polyunsaturated fatty acids are oxidized. Vitamin E protects other oxygen-sensitive compounds—vitamin A, for example—from oxidation.

Vitamin E also functions as an antioxidant in foods. The vitamin E in vegetable oils helps to keep them from being oxidized and becoming rancid. Frequently the vitamin is added to foods as a preservative because of its antioxidant properties.

Vitamin E may have other functions, but none has been clearly established as yet.

Deficiency of Vitamin E

In animals used in laboratory experiments symptoms of vitamin E deficiency are seen in the nervous, circulatory, and vascular system, and in the muscles and reproductive organs, but symptoms of deficiency are not the same in all animal species. The studies are complicated also because a few of the symptoms can be prevented by adding the

Vitamin E (Tocopherol)

inorganic element selenium (one of the trace minerals) to the animals' diets. The amount and kind of fat in the diet affects the rate of development and the severity of vitamin E deficiency.

In humans, however, it seems almost impossible to induce a vitamin E deficiency. Because the body has a reserve supply of vitamin E, only months or years of low vitamin E intake can deplete the storehouse. In an experiment conducted at Elgin State Hospital in Elgin, Illinois, test subjects were fed diets low but not completely lacking in vitamin E—some for as long as six years.[1,2] The results showed that the concentration of vitamin E in the blood gradually decreased until, after 20 months, it was about half the level of that in subjects fed the same diet with added vitamin E. Substitution of corn oil (with vitamin E removed) for lard in the diet caused a further decrease of vitamin E in the blood just as it had in experimental animals. The only other effect to appear as a result of the low vitamin E diet was a slight increase in the fragility of the red blood cells. No serious symptoms of vitamin E deficiency were seen in any of the subjects.

Evidence of mild vitamin E deficiency is sometimes seen when nutrients are poorly absorbed by the small intestine, a malfunction that occurs when bile is not produced by the liver or delivered to the small intestine where it is needed for the absorption of fats and fat-soluble vitamins. Liver and gall bladder diseases or damage to the small intestine also can decrease the absorption of vitamin E.

Vitamin E deficiency in newborn (especially premature) babies occurs because vitamin E is not transferred efficiently from the mother to the developing fetus. The most common symptom of this type of E deficiency is hemolytic anemia; the red blood cells are fragile and rupture, or hemolyze, at an unusually rapid rate. Administration of vitamin E to the babies in the amount normally obtained from human milk brings about a rapid recovery. It is important to add that the babies' vitamin deficiency usually is recognized and treated by doctors shortly after

Vitamin E (Tocopherol)

birth. (The E deficiency of the newborn has also been associated with milk formulas inadequate in the vitamin.)

Because these conditions are rare or easily recognized when they do occur, it can be assumed that enough vitamin E is supplied by the normal daily diet and that no need for a supplement is indicated.

Therapeutic Uses of Vitamin E

Supplemental vitamin E is advised only when there is evidence of a deficiency or risk of deficiency in a newborn baby or in a patient suffering from diseases that inhibit absorption of the vitamin.

Vitamin E therapy also may be beneficial in the relief of "intermittent claudication." Symptoms of this condition are pains in the leg muscles during walking or exercising. The pain goes away at rest. Damage or disease of the blood vessels in leg muscles is the apparent cause. Since there are a number of possible causes for leg pains and cramps, self-treatment with large doses of vitamin E is definitely *not recommended.*

Hazards and Toxicity of Vitamin E

Vitamin E appears comparatively safe. Many people have taken large doses of it for long periods of time without experiencing serious side effects. Experimental animals fed excessive amounts of vitamin E developed increased requirements for vitamins D and K, growth was stunted, and there were adverse effects on the thyroid gland. Although these conditions have not been seen in human subjects, some people taking more than 400 IU of vitamin E daily for long periods have suffered nausea, intestinal distress, fatigue, and other flu-like symptoms.

Claims and Controversy

A 1973 review of the benefits claimed for vitamin E listed

Vitamin E (Tocopherol)

60 conditions for which the vitamin had been recommended as a preventive, treatment or cure.[3] Among these were acne, aging, bee stings, liver spots on the hands, bursitis, diaper rash, frostbite, heart attacks, labor pains, miscarriage, muscular dystrophy, poor posture, sexual impotence, sterility, infertility, and sunburn. Some of these claims are based on findings from animal experimentation. But the gross vitamin deficiency that produces such symptoms as sterility and muscle deterioration in animals is not seen in human beings.

Adelle Davis, the late nutrition advocate, was a great supporter of vitamin therapy for many conditions.[4] Among them was vitamin E therapy for muscular dystrophy. She claimed that if vitamin E supplements were given before the disease "advanced" it could be quickly corrected. But her claim is scientifically unfounded. Muscular dystrophy in humans is a genetic disorder. It is illogical to expect a condition not caused by a vitamin deficiency to be cured by taking the vitamin in large doses.

Davis stated that careful studies indicated that adults usually require 140 to 210 IU of vitamin E daily and that 100 additional units should be taken for each tablespoon of oil in the diet. She recommended an intake of 600 to 1,600 IU of vitamin E daily. The available evidence discussed above shows 15 IU daily to be adequate.

Davis suggested that the normal adult diet does not contain sufficient amounts of vitamin E. She also contended that physicians often do not recognize the symptoms of a deficiency. This may be true since evidence of a lack of vitamin E is so rare that few physicians have seen cases.

Heart disease. The most widely publicized claim for vitamin E came from Drs. Wilfred and Evan Shute and their colleague, Dr. Albert Vogelsang. They reported that they were able to prevent and treat heart disease by using large amounts of vitamin E.[5,6] Their claim aroused excited interest in the medical and public communities when it appeared in 1946, but studies—conducted both in the

Vitamin E (Tocopherol)

United States and abroad—have not confirmed the report. Even without substantiating evidence, the Shutes continued to publish their beliefs about the benefits of vitamin E. The 1972 book, *Vitamin E for Ailing and Healthy Hearts* by Wilfred Shute and Harold Taub, included claims of their treatment of over 30,000 patients.[7] Acceptable supporting data were not provided, however.

Catharyn Elwood, in her book, *Feel Like A Million,* also perpetuates the myth of vitamin E supplements for healthy hearts.[8] And Richard A. Passwater cites the prevention of heart disease as a "speculative function" of vitamin E in his book, *Supernutrition—Megavitamin Revolution.*[9] The final stage of Passwater's step-by-step program recommends a daily intake of 800 IU of vitamin E along with large doses of other vitamins. As recently as 1977, investigators treated 48 patients with angina pectoris (one type of heart disease) with daily doses of 1,600 IU of vitamin E for six months.[10] No improvement in the patients' conditions was noted, and the claims remain unconfirmed.

Scarring and Aging. Vitamin E has also been touted as a wonder drug for smoothing out scars and blemishes and correcting dry, rough and aging skin. Face creams containing vitamin E were introduced and became popular in the late 1960s. In 1972 even a deodorant with vitamin E was produced and sold. But claims made for these products have not been substantially supported. The deodorant is no longer marketed.

Recent claims that vitamin E can delay aging—a process which involves many biochemical and physiological changes—are not easy to prove or disprove. Beginning at birth, aging is obviously a long-term event. So far, evidence from animal studies does not provide much hope for eternal youth from vitamin E supplements.

Air pollution. There are ongoing animal studies that suggest vitamin E may be useful in reducing lung damage caused by air pollution. The common air pollutants, ozone and nitrogen dioxide, apparently cause lung damage by oxidation reactions affecting the lung cells. Early experi-

Vitamin E (Tocopherol)

ments revealed that vitamin E-deficient animals were more susceptible to lung damage from these pollutants than animals receiving adequate amounts of the vitamin. It will take further testing to determine if vitamin E can protect people from air pollution.

Medical Consensus

The Advisory Panel on OTC (over-the-counter) vitamin and mineral drug products concluded that there is no proven indication for the therapeutic use of vitamin E as a single-ingredient OTC drug.[11] The Panel recommended that drug products containing only vitamin E not be allowed, and the FDA proposed a regulation to this effect. This opinion about vitamin E supplements classified as drugs should be equally applicable to products sold as "dietary supplements."

The Food and Drug Administration concluded its review of vitamin E claims by stating: "In summary, vitamin E has not been proven scientifically to have any of the miraculous effects being claimed for it. And the FDA sees no reason for persons in good health and eating a well-balanced diet to use a dietary supplement."[12]

CONSUMER GUIDE® magazine Opinion

There is no evidence of even marginal vitamin E deficiency in the American people. And, although taking large amounts of the vitamin (over 400 IU) seems comparatively safe, there is no proof that this is of any value. *Caution:* If you accept the unfounded claims for vitamin E and use them to diagnose and treat a physical condition yourself, the delay in getting proper medical treatment might have serious consequences.

Vitamin E Summary

Type of vitamin: Fat-soluble

Vitamin E (Tocopherol)

Where stored in the body: All body tissues; especially fatty tissues
Length of storage: Long-term (months to years)
History: Discovered in 1922; isolated in 1936
Food sources: Best food sources are vegetable oils: corn, cottonseed, soybean, and safflower. Other sources include wheat germ, whole-grain cereals, egg yolk, and liver.
Recommended Dietary Allowance: The RDA for women is 12 IU per day; for men, 15 IU per day.
Function: Vitamin E is an antioxidant which protects polyunsaturated fatty acids and other oxygen-sensitive compounds from undesirable oxidation.
Deficiency: Vitamin E deficiency is unknown in persons eating a usual mixed diet, but there is a risk of deficiency in persons with diseases that impair the absorption of nutrients in the small intestine and some risk in newborn (especially premature) babies.
Therapeutic uses: Physicians may recommend vitamin therapy to prevent or correct deficiencies associated with the above conditions.
Hazards and toxicity: Large doses can be used by most people without harmful effects. Flu-like symptoms in some individuals taking more than 400 IU daily over long periods (weeks to months) have occurred.
Claims and controversy: No scientific documentation exists for the prevention, treatment, or cure in humans of the diseases or conditions for which beneficial effects have been claimed.
CONSUMER GUIDE® magazine opinion: Unless your doctor specifically prescribes vitamin therapy to prevent or treat a deficiency you gain nothing by taking vitamin E supplements. *Do not self-treat any disease with vitamin E supplements or megavitamins.*

Vitamin K

The "k" in vitamin K was derived from the Danish word "koagulation," for blood clotting, and is used as the vitamin's designation because it precisely reflects its function in the human body.

History

The importance of a dietary factor in blood clotting was first recognized by the Danish scientist Henrik Dam. In 1929 he reported that chicks fed diets without a particular dietary factor had hemorrhages because their blood was slow to form the clots that are needed to control bleeding. The dietary factor, then called the "antihemorrhagic factor," turned out to be vitamin K.

Vitamin K

Food Sources of Vitamin K

Vitamin K includes not one but three compounds that have the same biologic activity. Two of these compounds occur naturally. The best source of vitamin K_1 is plants, especially green, leafy ones, and vitamin K_2 is produced by bacteria in animals which makes meat and dairy products good sources. Fruits, nonleafy vegetables, and cereals have only small amounts of the vitamin. Water-soluble vitamin K_3 is synthetic, and is a provitamin; that is, a substance the body can use to form the vitamin.

Dietary Requirements for Vitamin K

Vitamin K is synthesized in the human intestine from bacteria already present. Since no one knows how much of the vitamin the bacteria generate, estimates of dietary needs are difficult to make. A usual mixed diet in the United States, however, supplies from 300 to 500 micrograms (μg) of the vitamin each day, which is more than enough to meet dietary needs.

Function of Vitamin K

Vitamin K's only known biologic role is in the blood clotting mechanism, which involves the production of several substances. One of them, coagulation Factor II, will not be made in sufficient amounts unless the supply of vitamin K is adequate. When the supply is inadequate, coagulation of the blood is slow, bleeding may go unchecked, and the loss of blood may be serious.

Deficiency of Vitamin K

Vitamin K deficiency due to lack of the vitamin in the diet is unlikely. The vitamin is widely distributed in both plant and animal food sources; foods in the green vegetable, meat, and dairy classes usually will provide adequate amounts of

Vitamin K

the vitamin. Also, the natural forms of the vitamin are fat-soluble, so they are stored in the body to some extent and provide a reserve that may be tapped when necessary.

When a deficiency does occur, it most often affects newborn babies. Newborn, especially premature, infants have little vitamin K because the vitamin cannot easily pass from the mother to the fetus through the placenta before birth. And, for one to two days after birth, the baby's intestinal tract has no bacteria to create the vitamin. So until the vitamin is taken in with food or the vitamin K-producing bacteria take up residence in the intestine, the infant may have a vitamin K deficiency and a possible bleeding problem.

Vitamin K deficiency in adults is rare, but it may arise from liver or gall bladder disease or diseases of the intestinal tract that hinder absorption of fats and fat-soluble vitamins. And mild vitamin K deficiency may follow long-term use of oral antibiotics. If antibiotics are taken for an extended period of time, they may kill not only disease-causing bacteria but also the vitamin K-producing bacteria.

Therapeutic Uses of Vitamin K

Physicians commonly prescribe vitamin K therapy to prevent bleeding problems in newborns. And they use supplements to treat vitamin deficiency in people who, because of disease, cannot absorb the vitamin. Doctors also may give vitamin K supplements to patients who have been taking antibiotics for an extended period of time to prevent deficiency.

Sometimes, physicians prescribe large doses of vitamin K to people who are taking drugs that inhibit the action of the vitamin—for example, drugs used in the treatment of heart disease or of an ailment that creates a tendency toward too-easy blood clotting. These drugs lower the concentration of coagulation Factor II so the risk of clot

Vitamin K

production is reduced. But if the level of coagulation Factor II becomes too low, patients may start to bleed, so physicians must carefully monitor their patients and administer vitamin K to raise the level of coagulation Factor II if needed.

Hazards and Toxicity of Vitamin K

Treatment of vitamin K deficiency must be under the direction of a physician. Only a physician can determine an individual's need for the vitamin, and only a physician can guard against the adverse effects that may accompany vitamin K_3 therapy. (For example, too much supplemental vitamin K_3 can cause red blood cells to rupture and release compounds that accumulate in the blood and brain.) Vitamins K_1 and K_2 are relatively safe.

Because of the hazards of vitamin K therapy, the Food and Drug Administration prohibits the inclusion of vitamin K in multivitamin supplements and recommends that the vitamin be sold only by prescription. Still, some single-ingredient supplements contain as much as 100 μg of vitamin K_1.

CONSUMER GUIDE® magazine Opinion

We strongly advise against the use of vitamin supplements containing vitamin K. Treatment with vitamin K can be managed safely *only* under a physician's watchful eye.

Vitamin K Summary

Type of vitamin: Fat-soluble K_1 and K_2; water-soluble K_3 (a synthetic)
Where stored in the body: The body stores vitamins K_1 and K_2 to a certain extent in the liver.
History: Discovered in 1929
Food sources: Green, leafy vegetables; meats; and dairy products

Vitamin K

Recommended Dietary Allowance: No RDAs have been established; the usual mixed diet provides 300 to 500 micrograms—more than enough to meet dietary needs.
Function: To ensure normal blood clotting
Deficiency: Vitamin K deficiency may cause abnormal bleeding.
Therapeutic uses: Doctors prescribe vitamin K: to correct a deficiency caused by long-term use of oral antibiotics or by a disease that interferes with the absorption of the vitamin; to prevent a deficiency in newborns; and to reverse the effect of anticoagulant drugs when necessary.
Hazards and toxicity: Excess amounts of vitamin K_3 can cause red blood cells to rupture and release compounds that accumulate in the blood and the brain causing serious damage, especially in infants.
Claims and controversy: None
CONSUMER GUIDE® magazine opinion: We strongly advise against the use of supplemental vitamin K. Vitamin K therapy can be managed safely only when under the direction of a physician.

Vitamin Supplements

With all our knowledge of vitamins, these vital nutrients still seem shrouded in mystery. The idea that vitamins are endowed with almost miraculous powers persists. This mystery, combined with a misunderstanding about how vitamins work, leads many to believe that daily vitamin supplements are essential for good health.

People are concerned that our food supply is being robbed of its nutritional value and that it is difficult to get the required vitamins through our daily diets alone. Promoters of vitamin supplements feed this notion with expressions like "just to be sure you get all the vitamins you need." To

Vitamin Supplements

add to the confusion, vitamins—especially massive doses of them—are promoted for the prevention and cure of diseases totally unrelated to known deficiencies.

Vitamin supplements are available as liquids, capsules, or tablets and are either natural or synthetic. Some are chewable and fruit-flavored and some have time-release capabilities. Supplements may contain only one vitamin or as many as twelve. Many times a variety of nonvitamin substances are also present. The dosage of the vitamin varies widely from one supplement to another, from relatively low to extremely high quantities. This chapter will help you to weed through the tangle of data that continues to grow up around vitamins.

Vitamin Status—USA

Full-blown vitamin deficiency diseases are seldom seen in the United States today. Most practicing physicians have never seen a case of scurvy, beriberi, pellagra, or rickets. What diseases do occur can be traced to a deficiency usually caused by poverty, child abuse or neglect, ignorance or indifference about food selection, or to adoption of bizarre food habits. Although vitamin deficiencies rarely are seen, this doesn't necessarily mean that the nutrition and vitamin status of the population is completely satisfactory.

A dietary lack of a vitamin produces a continuum of effects. Body tissues lose any vitamin reserves they may have, biochemical and metabolic reactions that require the vitamin are adversely affected, and finally obvious symptoms of deficiency appear. The stages prior to development of readily apparent symptoms have been characterized as "subclinical deficiency." Subclinical deficiency may or may nor impair overall health, but it definitely represents a state of "nutritional risk."

The vitamin status of some 40,000 Americans of all ages was evaluated during the Ten-State Nutrition Survey (TSNS) between the years 1968 and 1970 and conducted

Vitamin Supplements

by the Nutrition Program of the United States Public Health Service. Most of the participants in the survey were from low-income populations.

The original plan for the survey did not include evaluation of status for all of the essential vitamins, and physical examinations did not reveal obvious symptoms of vitamin deficiency. But, blood and urine analysis showed that many of those included in the survey population were at "risk" levels. That is, they were in danger of developing vitamin deficiency. Mexican-Americans in Texas had a major problem with respect to vitamin A. Young people in general had unsatisfactorily low blood plasma vitamin A values. Riboflavin status was poor among blacks and among young people of all ethnic groups. The major nutrition problem, however, was that of iron intake and iron deficiency anemia. (Neither vitamin C nor thiamin levels appeared to be major problems.)

The dietary studies tended to correlate with the findings of clinical and biochemical examinations for the same study population. For example, individuals with low blood plasma vitamin A concentrations also consumed relatively low amounts of the vitamin. Analysis of food intake records indicated that unsatisfactory nutritional status was more a function of the quantity of food available than of the quality of the diets. In other words, many people simply did not get enough to eat. This related to family income—the lower the income, the poorer the status.

Consequently, efforts to improve nutritional status of the American people should concentrate on providing more food. Although nutrition problems in low-income populations are largely due to economics, some improvement might be stimulated by education programs designed to help people make better food choices and to use their food dollars more wisely.

In 1971-72 the National Center for Health Statistics conducted its first Health and Nutrition Examination Survey (HANES) with objectives and procedures similar to those of the TSNS. In the HANES study, however, the

Vitamin Supplements

more than 10,000 people who were surveyed represented a broader cross-section of the American population. Participants were not concentrated in the low-income group. Not all of the results of this survey have been released, but those available are in general agreement with findings of the TSNS. Plans to monitor the nutritional status of the American population by repeated surveys of this type will continue to add to our growing knowledge of the national nutritional picture.

What is confirmed by these and continuing studies is that the vitamin status of some segments of our population is not completely satisfactory. The reasons are largely related to a variety of socioeconomic factors. Better nutritional status can be expected only when these contributing factors are recognized and dealt with satisfactorily.

Unfortunately, findings from TSNS and HANES surveys have been used in grossly misleading ways to promote the sale of vitamin supplements. Advertisements for vitamins include the statements: "Surveys show that a large number of people in our country don't get all the vitamins they need." The implication is that these people need vitamin supplements. Statements of this sort are made with no qualification or reference to the factors responsible for the low vitamin intakes. Any money spent on vitamin supplements by people with limited incomes could be better used to buy ordinary foods that contain the vitamins. Many nutrition problems in this country could be corrected by more food or by better food selection.

Who Needs Vitamin Supplements?

"Do *I* need vitamin supplements?" you may ask. But no firm answer is possible without a thorough investigation of your individual eating habits, life-style and all the other factors which affect the intake and use of the nutrients in your daily diet.

Vitamin deficiencies due primarily to a faulty diet or

Vitamin Supplements

appearing as the result of some disease condition should be treated with appropriate vitamin supplements. In either case diagnosis of deficiency should be made by a qualified physician. If precipitated by disease, the disease must be treated. During treatment and before cure is complete, supplementary vitamins may be prescribed. Treatment is conducted on an individual basis with complete knowledge of the disease and its effect on vitamin status.

Vitamin therapy for treatment of diseases unrelated to vitamin deficiency is effective in only a few instances. Unfortunately, the consumer is constantly exposed to promotion of vitamins as wonder drugs. Such promotion is often motivated more by money than by health concerns and unfettered by constraints imposed by medicine, science, or ethics.

Authors of books, guests on talk-shows, and writers of newspaper columns cannot ethically diagnose or prescribe treatment for disease. This task remains with the medical profession.

Prevention through use of vitamin supplements of diseases not caused by deficiencies is extremely difficult to prove or disprove. A person who takes vitamins and does not develop a certain disease often attributes his good fortune to the supplement. This is not proof, however.

Many people take vitamin supplements as a type of "nutrition insurance." They don't know for sure what their vitamin status is, and they don't really know the amount of vitamins present in the foods they eat, so they use vitamin supplements just to be sure.

Nutritionists generally agree that people can get all the vitamins they need from foods, provided they get enough of the right kinds of foods. Nutritionists, however, usually will not quarrel with the use of vitamins for "insurance" *if the supplement is one in which the vitamins are supplied in amounts approximating the Recommended Dietary Allowances (RDAs).* Nutrition authorities do not support the use of supplements containing megadoses of vitamins.

If you want to know if you need to take vitamin

Vitamin Supplements

supplements, CONSUMER GUIDE® magazine recommends that you consult your physician for competent evaluation of your vitamin status.

Vitamins and Dieters

Diets including enough food of different kinds usually supply vitamins in sufficient quantity. There are situations, however, which do cause some concern. Many people in this country are trying to lose weight and follow widely publicized weight-reduction diets in which food choices are limited. These weight-reduction diets often do not include the "Basic Four." (See the chapter entitled Eating Right Is Up to You.) Even without restricting the types of food eaten, cutting down on calories results in less food being eaten. Consequently, there is concern that vitamin intakes may be less than desirable among calorie-conscious people. Vitamin supplements may provide a hedge against deficiency for these people.

Vitamins and the Elderly

There is growing concern that the vitamin status of elderly people may be threatened by inadequate or inappropriate diets. Older people need fewer total calories than younger adults because they are generally less active. The elderly cut down on the amount of food eaten in order to avoid becoming overweight. Many also do not eat well for reasons related to economics, loneliness, physical handicaps, and reduced mobility. While vitamin supplements may be useful as insurance for older people in the population, the better solution is the combination of an adequate diet and better eating habits.

Vitamins for Pregnant Women, Infants, and Children

Vitamin supplements are almost routinely prescribed for pregnant women and for infants. Pregnancy increases the

Vitamin Supplements

need for vitamins. Vitamin supplements provide assurance that requirements will be met during pregnancy, but actual need is not always evaluated.

A breast-fed infant may not get enough vitamin D from his mother's milk. And cow's-milk formulas supply only small amounts of vitamin C. Consequently, pediatricians frequently prescribe a supplement containing vitamins A, D, and C for babies. Usually in liquid form, the supplement can be added to formulas, soft foods, or squirted directly into the mouth. It should be used only according to directions to avoid intake of excessive amounts.

Chewable vitamin supplements are popular for young children. They are available in a variety of flavors, sizes and shapes—animals, monsters, and popular cartoon characters—to interest the child in taking them. This very appeal, their candy-like appearance and taste, has caused concern about possible overuse of the supplements. Even though they are sold with child-proof bottle caps, accidents can happen. Reports of serious poisoning from consumption of a large number of chewable supplements point up the potential danger.

Small children may have difficulty in swallowing tablets or capsules; they usually can learn to do so with parental guidance and patience. Chewable vitamins offer an easy solution, but extreme care must be exercised in the handling and storage of these supplements. These, as well as any other vitamin-mineral supplements or drugs, must be kept out of the reach of children.

Children, like adults, can get all the vitamins they need from a properly planned diet. Nutritionists emphasize the importance of introducing children to a variety of foods and of encouraging early development of good eating habits. Vitamin supplements should not be used as an excuse for allowing your child to develop bad eating habits.

Supplements Not Substitutes

Some people think that as long as they take vitamin

Vitamin Supplements

supplements they don't need to worry about how they eat. Vitamin supplements should not be used as an excuse for dietary slothfulness. All essential nutrients must be supplied in adequate amounts to ensure good nutrition and good health. Nutrients are a team and vitamins are just one part of that team.

If you are concerned about whether or not you are getting all the vitamins you need, and choose to use a vitamin supplement as a form of "nutrition insurance" be sure to select a supplement that contains no more than 100 percent of the U.S. RDAs.

Checking the Label

The following table illustrates the kind of information included on the labels of vitamin supplements. The principal, or front panel, shows the trade name of the product, the name of the manufacturer, the number of tablets or capsules in the container, and the general nature of the supplement; in this case a multivitamin supplement. Other descriptive expressions that might appear on the front panels of supplement labels include: multivitamin/multimineral supplement; multiple vitamin with (or plus) iron; vitamin supplement with minerals; multivitamin—therapeutic; high potency vitamin formula; B-complex vitamins; and vitamins A, D, and C.

This label also shows for whom the product is intended—"For adults and children 4 or more years of age." This information may not always be on the front panel and may not be specifically stated elsewhere. (Statements of "intended use" are not usually shown on labels of single-vitamin supplements.)

The contents panel gives directions for use ("One Tablet Daily"). Then the vitamins in the supplement are listed, together with the amount of each in a daily dose expressed as "Percent of U.S. RDA." The amounts are also frequently shown with measures such as milligrams (mg), micrograms (μg or mcg) and international units (IU).

Vitamin Supplements

SAMPLE PORTIONS OF A VITAMIN SUPPLEMENT LABEL

Front Panel

VITA-SURE*
MULTIVITAMIN SUPPLEMENT

For adults and children
4 or more years of age

100 tablets

Wishing-You-Well Vitamin Company*

Contents Panel

One Tablet Daily

Vitamin	Quantity	Percent of U.S. RDA
Vitamin A	5,000 IU	100
Vitamin E	15 IU	50
Vitamin C	60 mg	100
Folic Acid	0.4 mg	100
Thiamin	1.5 mg	100
Riboflavin	1.7 mg	100
Niacin	20 mg	100
Vitamin B_6	2 mg	100
Vitamin B_{12}	6 μg	100
Vitamin D	400 IU	100
Pantothenic Acid	10 mg	100

Expiration date — July, 1981

*These names are used for purpose of illustration only. They are not meant to represent an actual product or company.

We recommend that you select a preparation that provides vitamins in amounts approximating 100 percent of the U.S. RDAs and avoid those with amounts in excess

Vitamin Supplements

of the U.S. RDAs. A supplement with a composition like the one illustrated would be a suitable choice.

You will note that 10 of the 11 vitamins in our sample are provided in amounts equal to 100 percent of the U.S. RDA. For vitamin E only 50 percent of the U.S. RDA is furnished. This is because U.S. RDAs were derived from the 1968 revision of the Food and Nutrition Board's Recommended Dietary Allowances when the adult RDA for vitamin E was 30 IU. The RDA was reduced to 15 IU in the 1974 revision. Therefore, 50 percent of the U.S. RDA for this vitamin is equal to 100 percent of the current RDA.

The label must also provide a list of ingredients (not shown). In many cases this list will give the chemical form of the vitamin or mineral present, plus substances which may have been used as fillers, binders, and coloring or flavoring agents. In some instances, especially for the so-called natural supplements, the ingredients list will contain the names of nonvitamin or non-nutrient compounds derived from the natural sources of the vitamins or minerals. There are supplements for which a different format is used. A section with the heading "other components" may appear instead of one identified as "ingredients." The list of vitamins and minerals plus the other

---

**SAMPLE PORTIONS OF A NATURAL
VITAMIN SUPPLEMENT LABEL**

Front Panel

MOTHER NATURE'S TABLEt
VITAMINS AND MINERALS
from NATURAL SOURCES
plus Additional
Natural Ingredients

100 Tablets

Be-Well Vitamin Companyt

Vitamin Supplements

Contents Panel

Directions: As a dietary supplement of the listed vitamins and minerals take six tablets daily. Each six (6) tablets contain:

Vitamin	Quantity	Percent of U.S. RDA*
Vitamin A (fish liver oil)	10,000 IU	200
Vitamin D (fish liver oil)	400 IU	100
Vitamin E	100 IU	333
Vitamin C (natural vitamin C and rose hips)	300 mg	500
Folic Acid	200 µg	50
Vitamin B_1 (yeast concentrate)	10 mg	666
Vitamin B_2 (yeast concentrate)	10 mg	588
Niacin (yeast concentrate)	10 mg	50
Vitamin B_6	1 mg	50
Vitamin B_{12} activity (cobalamin concentrate)	25 µg	417
Biotin	0.15 mg	50
Pantothenic Acid	5 mg	50
Choline (yeast concentrate)	24 mg	**

*U.S. Recommended Daily Allowance (U.S. RDA) for adults and children four or more years of age.
**No U.S. RDA has been established for this nutrient.

† *These names are used for purpose of illustration only. They are not meant to represent an actual product or company.*

components would together account for all of the ingredients.

An expiration date is shown on the sample label. This date provides assurance that at any time prior to that date the supplement will provide you with vitamins of the potency shown on the label. Look for it. If it doesn't appear on the label, do not buy the vitamins.

The table on these two pages depicts the label of a "natural" vitamin supplement. The front panel shows that it

Vitamin Supplements

is a vitamin-mineral supplement from natural sources. The vitamins and their amounts are listed for comparison with the previous illustration. The actual label for such a supplement would also include a similar list of the minerals, plus a list of ingredients or "other compounds."

The persons for whom this supplement is intended is suggested by the footnote noting which set of the U.S. RDAs was used to express quantity. This procedure is not as satisfactory as that used in the first example because it does not state that the supplement is specifically intended for this age group.

Some of the natural sources for some of the vitamins are shown as fish liver oil, yeast concentrate, and rose hips. The vitamins represent 50 to 666 percent of the U.S. RDAs. Choline is included in the list, although it is not recognized as a vitamin nor a dietary essential for humans. For this reason, no U.S. RDA has been established for choline.

A variety of sources such as yeast, dried liver, fish liver oils, wheat germ oil, and bone marrow are used to prepare natural supplements. It would probably be technically difficult to compound a supplement with exactly 100 percent of the U.S. RDA for all of the vitamins included. There is no reason to be concerned about the safety of a product with the composition shown. Vitamins at the highest potency levels are the water-soluble ones, for which there is little evidence of toxicity or adverse side effects even with high doses. (Excess amounts of water-soluble vitamins will, for the most part, quickly pass from the body.)

There is no evidence to prove that natural vitamins are in any way superior to synthetic vitamins although they may cost more. The label may suggest that you are getting more for your money when you buy natural supplements. However, many of the "extras" are not dietary essentials, and the higher amounts of vitamins have no known nutritional value. You are buying things you don't need.

Vitamin Supplements

How To Buy Vitamin Supplements

It is almost impossible to give a meaningful evaluation of the cost of vitamin supplements. And with respect to quality, no one brand can be recommended since compliance with federal regulations means that they are all pretty much alike. The cost of vitamin supplements varies widely from brand to brand, from one retail outlet to another, and with the number of daily doses per container.

As is true for most products, the cost per unit decreases with an increase in the number purchased. So the daily cost of a vitamin supplement will be less when packages with 250 to 500 tablets are purchased than when a bottle with only 60 tablets is bought. The cost per day of multivitamin supplements providing 100 percent of the U.S. RDAs ranges from about two cents to slightly more than five cents, depending upon the brand and the retail outlet. If you decide to use a vitamin supplement, check labels to identify those with only 100 percent of U.S. RDAs, then make your own cost comparison. Divide the cost per container by the number of daily doses (tablets, capsules, or liquid measures) to find the cost per day.

There are a number of supplements which, in addition to vitamins at 100 percent U.S. RDA level, also include iron in an amount equal to 100 percent U.S. RDA. These cost about one-half cent per day more than those containing only vitamins. The addition of other minerals or inorganic elements raises the price still more. Natural supplements, which usually contain both minerals and vitamins, may cost as much as 10 to 15 cents per day. (See the table at the end of this chapter for comparative contents and costs of several natural vitamin supplements.)

Mineral Supplements

Requirements for the essential minerals (see the chapter on minerals) can be met with a diet containing a variety of

Vitamin Supplements

foods of different classes, with the exception of the iron needs of girls and women. Surveys show that females consume considerably less than the recommended amount of this inorganic element. Iron-deficiency anemia is prevalent among pregnant women, especially those from low socioeconomic groups. Other studies indicate that a large proportion of the female population has little or no reserve amounts of body iron, even though they may not be anemic. To many experts, this condition represents nutritional risk.

Without a conscientous effort to include iron-rich foods—such as liver or highly fortified foods—in the diet, it is extremely difficult to get 18 mg of iron per day, the U.S. RDA for girls and women. There may be good reason, therefore, for iron supplementation. Note that there are definite hazards associated with high intakes of iron. We would suggest that you consult your physician about the desirability of taking supplemental iron.

The so-called macroelements—those needed in relatively large amounts—such as calcium, phosphorus, and magnesium, may be included in vitamin-mineral supplements but only in amounts in the order of 10 to 25 percent of the U.S. RDA. U.S. RDAs have not yet been established for all of the trace elements known or believed to be essential for humans and supplements do not furnish all essential trace elements.

Currently, the inorganic element zinc has received a great deal of attention from nutritionists. The expression "with zinc" is emphasized in the promotion of many vitamin-mineral supplements. Supplements of zinc alone are becoming widely available. Some nutritionists believe that zinc intakes may be marginal or borderline at best. There is no current evidence of widespread zinc deficiency in this country. Until recently, no one worried about zinc and little attention was given to evaluation of zinc status. The current promotion of zinc products may merely be a vitamin "trend." We cannot recommend the use of zinc supplements without medical supervision.

Vitamin Supplements

There is evidence that high intakes of certain minerals increase requirements for or adversely affect the utilization of others. Because of the complementary work of vitamins and minerals there is potential for undesirable imbalances among nutrients when large amounts of a single nutrient are consumed. Until more is known about such interactions, we must advise against the use of any single-nutrient supplement if you don't first receive medical advice.

Vitamin Supplements

COMPOSITION OF SELECTED NATURAL VITAMIN SUPPLEMENTS

Percent U.S. RDA in amount recommended for daily use

	Solotron Natural Sales Co.	Prevention Natural Sales Co.	Nutri-Time Vital Foods	Organex Nature Food Centers	Master Formula Bioorganic Brand, Inc.	Mega-One
Vitamin A	200	200	500	200	200	200
Vitamin D	100	100	250	100	100	100
Thiamin (B_1)	1666	666	1200	400	400	3333
Riboflavin (B_2)	1470	588	1058	705	705	2941
Pyridoxine (B_6)	1250	50	630	6	3	2500
Vitamin B_{12}	1666	417	300	250	250	833
Vitamin C	250	500	500	333	333	500
Vitamin E	83	333	100	33	166	1000
Niacin	500	50	250	15	10	250
Pantothenic Acid	500	50	300	1	1	500
Folic Acid	25	50	—	—	*	100
Biotin	7	50	4	—	*	17

Vitamin Supplements

COMPOSITION OF SELECTED NATURAL VITAMIN SUPPLEMENTS

	Solotron Natural Sales Co.	Preventron Natural Sales Co.	Nutri-Time Vital Foods	Organex Nature Food Centers	Master Formula Bioorganic Brand, Inc.	Mega-One
	Milligrams in amount recommended for daily use					
Inositol	25	36	120	36	8	50
Choline	150	24	240	5	6	50
Rutin	25	30	34	30	20	—
p-Aminobenzoic acid	25	40μg	30	—	*	50
Bioflavonoids	25	30	34	—	50	—
Hesperidin	—	25	—	25	25	—
Minerals	yes	yes	yes	yes	yes	no
Cost per recommended daily amount	10¢ (1/day)	18¢ (6/day)	30¢ (6/day)	11.7¢ (6/day)	11.7¢ (6/day)	20.4¢ (2/day)

Information not available

The costs per day of vitamin supplements listed in this table were based on midwest prices in May 1979 and do not reflect a national average.

Megavitamin Therapy

Can massive doses of vitamin C prevent or treat the common cold? Are large amounts of niacin effective in controlling schizophrenia? Will upping your vitamin E intake protect you against heart disease?

Today, people are bombarded with claims for miracle cures by "multimegavitamin" therapy promoters who claim that vitamin supplements (containing several thousand percent of the U.S. RDA for some vitamins) are effective in treating any number of physical and mental disorders. These claims stubbornly stand without controlled clinical trials to hold them up. The effectiveness of such huge quantities of supplements to prevent or treat disease that is unrelated to vitamin deficiency has not been substantiated.

Megavitamin Therapy

Still, promotion of megavitamin therapy probably will continue unchallenged because the Food and Drug Administration (FDA) no longer has the authority to regulate the potency or composition of most vitamin products sold as "dietary supplements." For almost 15 years, the FDA tried to develop rules and regulations to govern the composition and labeling of vitamin-mineral supplements. It contended that regulations would eliminate the confusion that exists when consumers are confronted with the vast array of supplements which vary both qualitatively and quantitatively. Proposed regulations were designed to protect consumers against the hazards of taking excessive amounts of nutrients; to provide uniform and accurate information on labels; and to require scientifically rational amounts and combinations of the substances in dietary supplements.

In keeping with these aims and intentions, the FDA published a number of "proposals of rule making." But each time it did, the health food industry raised loud objections. The health food industry took its case to Congress, and in 1976 the President approved the act (commonly referred to as the Proxmire amendment) that stripped the FDA of its authority to regulate the composition of vitamins and minerals in dietary supplements. The FDA continued its efforts to limit the amounts of vitamins A and D in supplements by requiring supplements with excessive quantities of these vitamins to be sold only by prescription. But in 1977 the New York State Court of Appeals ruled that the FDA did not have the authority to even do this.

These legislative and judicial actions have opened the door to unrestrained marketing of high-potency vitamin supplements and the proliferation of books that advocate their use. In one of these books Richard Passwater supports the use of megavitamins by arguing against the Recommended Dietary Allowances (RDAs). He says:

> There is no scientific method that predicts the proper amount of vitamins that *you* require.

Megavitamin Therapy

Minimum daily requirements (MDR) and recommended daily allowances (RDA) are thought to be indications of need by many, but they aren't. First of all, MDRs and RDAs are changed every time the RDA committee of the National Academy of Sciences meets to establish them. Second, they are based on short-term animal studies, and aren't reliable even for the animals. . . . But the most important reason why MDR and RDA are meaningless to *you* is that they represent the levels of vitamins required to prevent immediate *recognizable* deficiencies in the *average* animal or person. . . . They do not seriously consider differences in life-style, environment, height, weight, occupation, temperament, emotional stress, illness, metabolic error, bad habits, activity, and the like, even though they claim to do so. They consider only the lowest nutrient level required to keep the idealized nonexistent "reference man," who is supposed to be the average healthy person, free from signs of deficiencies. You deserve better.[1]

Passwater is correct when he states that "there is no scientific method that predicts the proper amount of vitamins that *you* require." Individuals vary in their requirements for vitamins. He is not correct, however, when he says that the RDAs fail to consider these variables. As the Food and Nutrition Board explains: "The Recommended Dietary Allowances are the levels of intake of essential nutrients considered, in the judgment of the Food and Nutrition Board on the basis of available scientific knowledge, to be adequate to meet the known nutritional needs of practically all healthy persons. . . ."[2]

Passwater's mention of the minimum daily requirements (MDR) for vitamins and minerals refers to the Food and Drug Administration's guidelines for labeling that were established in 1941 and slightly revised in 1957. MDRs were not intended to be used as standards for dietary

Megavitamin Therapy

evaluations. They were based on the best scientific evidence available at the time. But today, they are outdated and have been replaced by the U.S. RDAs (see the chapter entitled Eating Right Is Up to You).

In his first criticism of MDRs and RDAs, Passwater implies that changes in the theses over the years must in some way invalidate them. But change is not necessarily bad. Since the early 1940s, when the RDAs originated, the science of nutrition has advanced tremendously. Much has been learned about the nutrient needs of the human body. Nutrition is not a static science, and as the knowledge of nutrition grows, the RDAs change.

Passwater's second criticism is unfounded. RDAs have not been established on the basis of animal studies alone. Preceding chapters cite many examples of experimental studies with human volunteers. And findings from such experiments are used by the Food and Nutrition Board to arrive at the recommended allowances.

As the Food and Nutrition Board states, "RDAs should not be confused with requirements. . . . RDAs (except for energy) are estimated to exceed the requirements for most individuals, and thereby ensure that the needs of nearly all are met."[2] Thus, RDAs *do not* represent "the levels of vitamins required to prevent immediate *recognizable* deficiencies" as Passwater suggests. The Board further states that "RDAs . . . . do not take into account special needs arising from infections, metabolic disorders, chronic diseases, or other abnormalities that require special dietary treatment. These must be considered as unique clinical problems that require individual attention."[2] The Board does not claim that RDAs are suitable for all regardless of differences in life-style, environment, height, weight, occupation, temperament, emotional stress, illness, metabolic error, bad habits, activity and the like.

Promoters of megavitamin therapy often begin with false premises and misinterpretations of the RDAs. In its review of available information, the FDA Advisory Panel on Vitamin and Mineral Drug Products for Over-the-Counter

Megavitamin Therapy

Human Use found no scientifically sound evidence to support the unrestrained use of vitamin products with high dosages.[3]

Despite scientific evidence that indicates there is no benefit but there is possible hazard associated with megavitamin therapy, the claims go on. The last stage of Passwater's Supernutrition program recommends the daily use of: two high-potency vitamin-mineral tablets; two high-potency B-complex tablets (or six regular B-complex tablets); three vitamin C tablets (1,000 mg each); four vitamin E capsules (200 IU each); and one mineral tablet.[1]

Passwater emphasizes the need for blood tests and a checkup by a physician before starting the program and again after 12 weeks. He provides instructions, however, for those who cannot see a doctor. During the 12-week interval, he guides the initiate to ever-increasing doses of vitamins according to the results of a self-administered questionnaire. But someone who answers "yes" to questions about the presence of certain symptoms (dizziness or fainting spells, chronic cough, hemorrhoids, painful menstruation, tender breasts, tightness in the chest, shortness of breath, or prostate trouble) should see a physician—not move up a step on the Supernutrition ladder.

Passwater's approach, and others like it, encourage self-treatment of diseases that require medical attention. And the potential health hazards of delaying proper treatment should be evident.

Some people may be able to take megadoses of some vitamins and get a psychological "lift" but no serious adverse effects. But knowledge about the safety or tolerance of massive doses of vitamins is still incomplete. And evidence of potential hazard associated with large doses of vitamins is growing.

When promoters of megavitamin therapy raise false hopes, they are little better than hawkers at a frontier medicine show. In the book *New Hope for Incurable Diseases,* Drs. E. Cheraskin and W.M. Ringsdorf, Jr.

Megavitamin Therapy

recommend megavitamin therapy and other dietary changes to combat diseases for which there is no known cure.[4] The authors, both members of the Department of Oral Medicine at the University of Alabama, Birmingham, were criticized by a colleague at the university. Dr. C.E. Butterworth, Professor of Medicine and Director of the Nutrition Program, found that the book contained misleading and erroneous statements and lacked sound scientific support for its claims. Dr. Butterworth added: "But it is cruel to raise false hope under any pretense. In my opinion, the book raises nothing but false hopes."[5]

Those who believe in megavitamin therapy may develop serious guilt feelings when they think they might have protected a loved one from serious disease—had they "only known" sooner. Adelle Davis made the unsupported claim that crib deaths could be prevented by breast-feeding and vitamin E.[6] For a family who has lost a child to this mysterious malady, this statement can only bring despair.

Samuel Valsrub, M.D., writing in the October 17, 1977 issue of the *Journal of the American Medical Association,* summed up the medical opinion of megavitamin therapy: "Not only is it an insult to the intelligence and an injury to the pocketbook, it is also a threat to health."[7]

Minerals

Almost 90 percent of the 103 known elements have been detected in living organisms—plants and animals. Although not all are essential, minerals exist throughout nature—in water and soils, in plants, and in animals that eat the plants.

The body uses minerals for many purposes. They help regulate biochemical reactions and control muscle movements. Electrical impulses would not travel along nerve pathways without minerals. Your blood could not transport oxygen and waste products such as carbon dioxide without minerals. Your bones would become weak and easily broken if it weren't for minerals. Minerals are found in every cell of the body and are involved in one way or

Minerals

another with almost everything your body does.

One way to group minerals is by their concentration in the body. Those present in large amounts are called the macroelements and include calcium, chlorine, magnesium, phosphorus, potassium, and sodium. Present in smaller amounts are the trace minerals or microelements. Copper, chromium, cobalt, fluorine, iodine, iron, manganese, molybdenum, selenium and zinc are all trace minerals. The functions of these elements are known.

A third group of minerals are the trace minerals whose functions are unknown. These minerals include aluminum, boron, cadmium, nickel, silicon, tin, and vanadium. They are found in the body in small quantities.

There may be other minerals in the body that haven't been discovered. Some trace minerals are present in such small quantities that only recently have tests been developed to detect them. New procedures and tests may need to be developed before additional minerals are found.

Because a certain mineral is known to be present in your body does not necessarily mean that it serves any useful function. Examples of this include the minerals aluminum, boron, and cadmium. No one knows for sure what these minerals do, or if they do anything at all.

Many of the minerals, if taken in large amounts, will interfere with your body's use of other minerals. Cadmium, for example, may interfere with your body's use of copper and zinc. Zinc, in turn, may conflict with the function of still other minerals. (Zinc is currently widely promoted as a dietary supplement.)

On the following pages, we introduce each mineral and discuss how it functions within the body. Because the amounts of minerals needed to keep the body healthy are small and readily available in the normal diet, we do not recommend that you take mineral supplements or vitamin supplement products containing minerals. Only a physician can determine and supervise the treatment of a mineral deficiency.

Minerals

Calcium and Phosphorus

Calcium is the most common mineral in your body and forms two percent of the entire body weight. It is important for normal structure and strength of bones and teeth, and about 99 percent of the calcium in your body is located there. It is essential for blood clotting, and it regulates the action of many enzymes in the body. Muscle contraction and relaxation depend on calcium. Calcium helps to control the amount of fluids that pass through the walls of your body's cells. It is involved in the transmission of electrical impulses along nerve pathways.

Rickets is caused by a vitamin D deficiency. Calcium is not absorbed, so the bones cannot develop normally. Leg bones are especially vulnerable, and without calcium the bones become weakened and bowed. Calcium, along with large doses of vitamin D are given to correct this situation.

Also, in a multiple vitamin supplement calcium is usually given to pregnant women to allow for the growth needs of the unborn child.

It is impossible to discuss calcium without also including a discussion of phosphorus. They exist in the body in a 2:1 ratio, and they work together. (About one percent of the body's total weight is phosphorus.)

About 80 percent of all phosphorus is used for bone and tooth formation. The rest is involved in the metabolism of each of the body's cells. Energy is stored in the "P" (for phosphate) in "ATP" (adenosine triphosphate)—the substance used by muscles as fuel. Phosphorus, as phosphate, combines with sugars in the chain of reactions to produce energy. Phosphorus also reacts with certain fatty substances in the body to promote their distribution in the blood. Each of these reactions is, in one way or another, involved in providing fuel to keep your body going.

The major sources of calcium are milk and dairy products which supply three-quarters of the calcium in the American diet. Foods high in protein are the best source of phosphorus. Meat, fish, poultry, eggs, and cereal products

Minerals

are the major sources in usual mixed diets.

If you eat balanced meals that contain some dairy products, you will receive enough calcium and phosphorus. If you do not or cannot drink milk or eat other dairy products, you should consume extra nondairy foods that are rich in calcium.

Chloride

Chlorine gas, used as a poison and a disinfectant, is a noxious, greenish-yellow gas. The chlorine that is useful to the human body is a different form of the same element called "chloride." It is the other part of table salt—sodium chloride.

Chloride is important in maintaining the water and acid-base balance in the body. It is a component of stomach acid. This acid is usually referred to as hydrochloric acid but it could also be called hydrogen chloride.

Depletion of body sodium or potassium is accompanied by loss of chloride. People who have vomited a great deal also may have lost a large amount of the mineral. Diarrhea lasting more than three days also may cause chloride depletion.

Chloride and sodium occur together in foods. Salt is a major source of chloride.

Magnesium

Two-thirds of the body's magnesium occurs in bone. The remaining magnesium is found in all cells throughout the body. Magnesium regulates various enzyme reactions, including those that permit the body's cells to use sugars for fuel.

Magnesium is needed to prevent muscle spasms and nervous system disorders that occur as a result of magnesium depletion. Magnesium is also used to treat deficiencies of the mineral itself, which occur in kidney disease, malabsorption syndromes, and alcoholism with

Minerals

malnutrition. Treatment in these situations is usually done intravenously, not orally.

Even in large amounts, magnesium is not toxic for persons with normal kidney function. Magnesium-containing preparations (e.g., Phillips' Milk of Magnesia laxative and antacid) are used as laxatives but overuse of magnesium may cause diarrhea. Conversely, magnesium may be prescribed, along with copious amounts of water, when severe states of prolonged diarrhea or when dehydration has occured.

The major food sources of magnesium include whole grains, dried beans and peas, soy beans, cocoa, and nuts.

Potassium

Potassium is vitally important to the maintenance of good health. The usual diet contains adequate amounts (2 to 6 grams per day) of the mineral.

Potassium is available in liquid or tablet preparations. Some products used as salt substitutes are also sources of potassium. In this form potassium looks and tastes almost like ordinary table salt, which contains sodium.

There are important differences in the function of potassium and sodium. For example, sodium is an important part of the body fluids found outside the cell. Potassium is found primarily inside the body's cells. Potassium is necessary for nerve conduction and muscle contraction and is important in carbohydrate and protein metabolism. And potassium helps in the regulation of the acid-base balance of the body.

Abnormally low or high potassium levels in the body may occur in disease conditions which interfere with the excretion or retention of the mineral. The underlying cause must be treated medically and the body potassium returned to normal with potassium therapy. Healthy people with normal kidney function do not develop dietary deficiency of potassium, nor are they harmed by high intakes of the mineral.

Minerals

Too much potassium could be dangerous in some persons and may cause nausea and vomiting. Consult your physician before you begin taking potassium.

It has been estimated that adults need about 2.5 g of potassium each day. The mineral is so widely distributed in legumes, whole grains, fruits, vegetables, and meats that a deficiency is unlikely in healthy persons eating a variety of foods. Apricots, avocados, bananas, cherries, orange juice, and tomatoes are especially rich in potassium.

Sodium

Sodium is known to most people as a part of common table salt, which is called sodium chloride. It is also a component of sodium bicarbonate, or baking soda.

Sodium is present chiefly in body fluids. It and water move around the body together. Sodium is readily absorbed from the intestine and is easily excreted by the kidneys. This means that most people use up sodium at a fairly high rate. Sodium is important in the maintenance of the body's acids and bases, and in regulating the body's water balance, and muscle and nerve action.

Many experts believe that high sodium intakes may be a factor in the cause of high blood pressure, but this may be true only for persons with a genetic susceptibility to this condition. At any rate, many people with high blood pressure are told to limit their sodium intake.

A major source of sodium is salt (sodium chloride) used in the processing, the home preparation, and flavoring of foods. Processed foods that are high in sodium include nuts and crackers with added salt, cured meats (e.g., ham, bacon), luncheon meats, brined pickles and olives, canned vegetables, and condiments (e.g., ketchup, mustard).

Cobalt

Cobalt occurs only in minute amounts in the human body, although it is quite widely distributed in nature. Its only

Minerals

known function is as a constituent of vitamin B_{12}, which is essential for the formation of red blood cells and to the treatment of pernicious anemia, a disease caused by the inability of the body to absorb vitamin B_{12}. Cobalt is of no value in the treatment of this disease, however, and no deficiency of cobalt is known to exist. The only known need for this element is for that contained in vitamin B_{12}.

Copper

Copper is closely related to iron. These two minerals have complementary functions in the body, and copper apparently helps the absorption of iron. Copper and iron are both involved in the production of energy. Copper-containing enzymes are essential for the synthesis of the myelin sheath of nerve fibers, the incorporation of iron into hemoglobin, the synthesis of a pigment in the skin, and in the formation of connective tissues.

Copper is so widely distributed and so little is required that a deficiency state is unknown. (There is evidence, however, that relatively low levels of copper intake may cause adverse effects; and the maximum safe level is not known.) Some people think there may be some connection between copper and arthritis, but so far no such relationship has been proved.

Fluorine

Fluorine (a gas) is found in the bones and teeth in the form of fluoride. In teeth it functions to provide protection against decay. And there is growing evidence that fluorine may play a role in maintaining bone structure and strength.

Most foods contain only small amounts of fluorine, although teas contain fairly large quantities. Seafoods are fair sources. Small fish (such as sardines) that are eaten with the bones are good sources. The addition of a fluorine salt (fluoride) to drinking water has resulted in a significant reduction in the prevalence of tooth decay.

Minerals

High intakes of fluorine may have adverse effects on both the bones and teeth. In localities where the drinking water is naturally high in fluoride, the teeth of the people living there became mottled, that is they developed black or brown spots. The amount of fluoride added to drinking water to decrease tooth decay is considerably less than the amount known to cause mottling.

Iodine

Iodine is a burgundy-colored solid that evaporates to form a purple vapor. The only known function of iodine in the body is to combine with an amino acid tyrosine to form thyroid hormones (thyroxine and triiodothyronine). These hormones control the overall body metabolism. When the thyroid gland is overactive, excess amounts of the hormones are produced leading to hyperthyroidism. Hypothyroidism is the result of inadequate hormone production by the thyroid gland.

When solid iodine is dissolved in alcohol, the solution is called iodine tincture and is used as an antiseptic. When iodine is combined with sodium or potassium the product is called an "iodide" (for instance, sodium iodide). These are white solids which are used as expectorants for colds or coughs or in the treatment of certain thyroid diseases.

Since seafood is a rich source of iodine, persons who live near the ocean are unlikely to become iodine deficient. Those who live inland get a similar benefit by using iodized salt and because the free distribution of food products across the country bring fresh coastal products inland.

Relatively large daily doses (20 mg to 4 g) of iodine over four months produced no toxicity. Some people are apparently sensitive to excess iodine and high intakes may cause adverse side effects in such persons.

Iron

Your requirements for iron are pressed upon you each day

Minerals

by radio and television commercials which stress the "importance of taking adequate daily iron." The ads tell you that you will have a better complexion, more energy and pep, and will be healthier if you take a product containing iron. Without a doubt, iron is the most publicized mineral; and because of this is also the most overused.

The body's need for iron was known many centuries ago. Early doctors recommended that pieces of iron be allowed to rust, then the rust soaked off and drunk. Since iron metal was hard and strong, iron was believed to give the body strength and durability.

Iron serves two primary purposes. It forms the central part of the hemoglobin of the red blood cells. Hemoglobin carries oxygen to all cells of the body and transports carbon dioxide to the lungs to be exhaled. Iron further functions as a vital part of many enzyme reactions. It is an essential component of the chain of reactions producing energy.

Almost everyone has heard of iron deficiency anemia. Although there may be no symptoms in mild cases of this deficiency, definite problems appear in more severe forms. The person becomes weak and easily fatigued, is short of breath, and may have uncomfortable heart palpitations (rapid heartbeat that causes "thumping" in the chest). Mild exercise may cause severe chest pain resembling a heart attack. The skin and lips lack color or glow. The nail beds appear blue or gray, and the nails become brittle and deformed. (Before you self-diagnose your own "tiredness" or "shortness of breath" as an iron deficiency anemia, consider the more probable causes—poor dietary habits and insufficient exercise.)

Iron deficiency anemia is characterized by a deficiency of hemoglobin. It can be caused by an inadequate supply of iron in the diet, loss of blood, impaired absorption of the mineral, or frequent pregnancies.

Of all the minerals commonly found in vitamin-mineral preparations, iron is the most potentially toxic. If a person accidentally swallows several iron tablets or capsules or

Minerals

supplements containing iron, significant toxic effects may result. Iron toxicity occurs most frequently in children because of the wide availability of tasty, chewable vitamin tablets that contain iron. (Also, the sugar-coated iron tablets look like candy.) Some adults taking daily doses of 200 mg or more of iron may experience nausea and abdominal cramps. Single doses in the range of 2 to 4 g may be lethal to children. It is estimated that one child dies every month from an overdose of iron. Death from iron is usually from the intense damage to the gastrointestinal tract or from damage to the liver.

Never take iron or a product containing iron without first checking with your physician. If you take an iron preparation without having a deficiency, symptoms may be masked. You may feel better, but your disorder may worsen.

Many forms of iron are used in supplemental products. Most products contain iron in the form of ferrous salts. The most common and cheapest form is called ferrous sulfate. Because of the bad taste, tablets of ferrous sulfate are usually sugar-coated.

Ferrous gluconate is another popular form of iron. These unpalatable tablets are also sugar-coated. Manufacturers claim that ferrous gluconate causes less gastrointestinal distress than ferrous sulfate or some other forms of iron. This claim, however, has not been proven scientifically. The effectiveness of coated and sustained-release iron supplements has not been well documented.

Liver is the best food source of iron. Other meats, whole-grain and enriched cereal products, dried peas and beans, nuts, shellfish, and green, leafy vegetables also are good sources of iron.

Manganese

The highest concentrations of manganese are found in the bones, liver, and certain glands (e.g., pituitary).

Manganese is a component of many enzymes. One of

Minerals

these is involved in the formation of urea, a waste product of protein metabolism. Manganese activates enzymes involved in the metabolism of carbohydrates, fats, and proteins.

There is no specific therapeutic use for manganese, so there is no reason to include it in vitamin-mineral products. Sufficient manganese is found in dietary items to prevent any manganese deficiency.

Manganese poisoning appears to be nonexistent except where people are exposed to industrial contamination. Miners who work with manganese ores inhale toxic amounts of manganese dust. The mineral deposits in their livers and brains and causes an ailment that resembles Parkinson's disease.

Whole-grain cereal products, nuts, dried peas and beans, coffee, tea, and green vegetables are good sources of manganese. Animal products are poor sources.

Molybdenum

Only minute amounts of this trace element are present in the body. Molybdenum is necessary for the function of several enzymes, and is possibly involved in iron metabolism. Little is known about its requirement in humans.

Good food sources of molybdenum include legumes (dried peas and beans), whole-grain cereal products, milk, leafy vegetables, and organ meats.

Selenium

Selenium is known to be a component of a specific enzyme which functions to maintain the structure of cell membranes. Dietary deficiency of selenium has been produced experimentally causing symptoms which are correctable when the element is restored to deficient diets. So selenium seems to be an essential nutrient for many species of animals. But proof of human need is not available; no symptoms or conditions which can be

Minerals

explained by selenium deficiency have been documented in humans. It is generally assumed, however, that selenium is an essential nutrient for man.

Human dietary requirements for selenium are not known. Since deficiency does not occur it can be assumed that usual, mixed diets provide adequate amounts.

In humans there is no evidence of selenium toxicity resulting from above-average dietary intakes of the element. This is true even in geographic areas where the soil and the plants grown there have unusually high selenium contents. Selenium toxicity has been seen in experimental animals fed diets containing large amounts of selenium. The maximum safe level of selenium intake by humans is not known.

In view of these facts, the widespread promotion and marketing of selenium-containing supplements cannot be justified. There is definitely no need for supplemental selenium, and overuse of selenium-containing supplements may yet be proven hazardous.

Zinc

Zinc is widely distributed in the body. It is found in the pancreas, liver, kidneys, lungs, muscles, bones, eyes, male sex glands, and sperm. The only microelement present in larger quantities than zinc is iron.

Zinc's functions in the body are not completely understood, but it is known to be necessary for enzymes involved in the transport and elimination of carbon dioxide and in protein digestion.

Zinc appears to play a role in insulin metabolism, in the metabolism of DNA and RNA (ribonucleic acid), and in the function of white blood cells.

Zinc deficiency may lead to delayed puberty and dwarfism. It usually occurs as a result of a disease condition and should be treated under medical supervision.

Therapeutically, zinc has been used successfully in the

Minerals

treatment of acrodermatitis enteropathica. This disease produces zinc deficiency because the mineral cannot be efficiently absorbed. Another experimental use of zinc compounds is in the attempt to speed the healing of wounds such as bed sores or diabetic ulcers. Supplemental zinc may speed up the rate of healing in patients who are deficient but apparently is of little benefit to nondeficient persons.

Single large doses (several grams) of zinc cause severe kidney damage. Little is known about the safety of the long-term use of supplements which may increase the level several times higher than the requirement. There is concern that excess zinc may adversely affect the absorption and metabolism of other minerals.

Zinc is widely distributed in nature; a dietary deficiency is unlikely. Oysters are the richest source of zinc. Meat, poultry, eggs, cheese, whole-grain cereals, and nuts are good sources.

The Body's Mineral Balance

The human body has finely tuned mechanisms for regulating its supply of the macromineral elements. For example, when excess amounts of sodium, potassium and chloride begin to accumulate, the body simply gets rid of them in the urine. When the body needs more calcium, the mechanism for absorbing this mineral becomes more efficient. A larger proportion of the mineral is absorbed from the diet than is the case when the body has an adequate supply.

For these reasons the human body can adapt to a wide range of dietary intakes of the macrominerals without the appearance of either deficiency symptoms or adverse effects. Only when the body's regulating mechanisms fail, as in disease conditions which interfere with the absorption, excretion, and retention of the minerals, will the body supply become either depleted or dangerously high.

For most of the trace minerals (microelements) there are

Minerals

no such precise mechanisms for controlling the amounts in the body. At least marginal dietary deficiencies of iron and zinc are seen in this country, because intakes are low and because these minerals are not efficiently absorbed. Iodine deficiency was common in certain regions of the country prior to the iodization of salt.

Because excess amounts of many trace minerals tend to accumulate in the body, high intakes of most trace minerals can be toxic or have adverse effects. For some of these the margin of safety—the difference between the amount needed by the body and the amount producing toxic or adverse effects—is not known. At best, extrapolation of knowledge can only be made from animal studies.

The quantity of trace elements in a daily dose of readily available mineral-containing supplements is within the limits of safety. But there may well be hazard associated with overzealous use of such supplements, and for the most part no benefit can be anticipated.

The Food and Drug Administration's Advisory Panel on Vitamin and Mineral Drug Products for Over-the-Counter Human Use concluded that the only minerals appropriate for inclusion in such products for prevention of deficiency were calcium, iron, and zinc. Since deficiencies of other minerals are rare or unknown or are secondary to disease conditions, there is no good reason for including minerals other than the three named in mineral drug products. The panel further concluded that no mineral supplement should be available as an OTC product if it is represented for the treatment of a deficiency. Mineral deficiencies should be managed by a physician, and if supplements are considered to be necessary they should be by prescription only.

CONSUMER GUIDE® magazine Opinion

No vitamin supplement containing minerals and no individual mineral supplement should be used to treat a real or suspected mineral deficiency without a physician's advice.

Minerals

MINERALS (INORGANIC ELEMENTS)

The following minerals are those macroelements and microelements (trace elements) that are essential or believed to be essential to human health. The chart contains some elements not previously covered in this chapter; these are minerals about which there is little known. Included in the following information is each mineral's function, the food sources, the human requirements, and the results of deficiency if known.

Mineral	RDA or Estimated Requirement for Adults	Food Sources	Deficiency
Macroelements			
Calcium: Almost all of the body's calcium is in bones and teeth; only one percent is in body fluids essential for blood clotting, muscle contraction, and transmission of nerve impulses.	RDA: 800 mg	Milk and dairy products are the best food sources. Green, leafy vegetables are good sources.	Caused only by low intakes, deficiency is extremely rare. It may occur secondary to vitamin D deficiency, adversely affecting bones and teeth.
Chloride: Components of stomach acid; with other elements helps to maintain acid-base balance in body fluids.	RDA not established	Chloride supplied by salt (sodium chloride) present in or added to foods.	Dietary deficiency does not occur in humans unless salt intake is severely restricted.

212

Minerals

Magnesium: Most of the body's magnesium is in bones; the remainder is inside body cells taking part in many enzyme reactions. Important for nerve and muscle function.	RDA: men: 350 mg; women: 300 mg	Dried peas and beans, nuts, whole-grain cereals, cocoa, and chocolate are the best food sources. Green, leafy vegetables are good sources.	Deficiency causes muscle tremors, weakness, behavioral disturbances. Usually seen only in disease conditions, e.g., alcoholism, kidney disease, malabsorption syndromes.
Phosphorus: Eighty percent of the body's phosphorus is in bones and teeth. Present in all cells as part of compounds vital for many reactions of metabolism; essential for energy production.	RDA: 800 mg	Milk, dairy products, meats, dried peas and beans, and whole-grain cereals are good sources. Fruits and vegetables have small amounts.	Dietary deficiency does not occur in humans. Deficiency may occur secondary to prolonged and excessive use of some antacids.
Potassium: Most of the body's potassium is present inside cells; very little is in body fluids. Helps to regulate acid-base and fluid balance; important for regulating muscle action and transmission of nerve impulses.	RDA not established; healthy adults need about 2.5 g per day.	Bananas, citrus fruits, carrots, green, leafy vegetables, potatoes, and tomatoes are rich sources. Whole-grain cereals, meats, and seafoods are good sources.	Deficiency usually seen only in disease conditions which cause excessive loss of body potassium.

Minerals

MINERALS (CONTINUED)

Mineral	RDA or Estimated Requirement for Adults	Food Sources	Deficiency
Sodium: Sodium is present in fluids outside of cells; only small amounts are found within cells. Sodium functions with chloride and potassium to regulate water and acid-base balance and to regulate muscle and nerve action.	RDA not established; intakes probably range from about 2.5 g to 7 g per day.	Sodium content of animal foods (meats, dairy products, eggs) higher than that of fruits, vegetables, and cereals. Main source is salt used in processing, preservation, and seasoning.	Dietary deficiency does not occur in humans. Excessive losses of body sodium in certain disease conditions may cause evidence of deficiency.
Microelements			
Chromium: Necessary for maintaining normal blood concentration of sugar (glucose).	RDA not established; the World Health Organization suggests 20 to 50 µg per day is needed to replace urinary losses.	Meats, especially liver, whole-grain cereals, and brewer's yeast are good sources. Availability from food varies widely.	Deficiency apparently causes disturbances in blood sugar metabolism. Marginal deficiency may exist during pregnancy, in diabetics, and in the elderly.
Cobalt: Functions only as integral part of vitamin B_{12}.	RDA not established; no need except as B_{12}.	Vitamin B_{12} present only in animal foods (meats, seafood, and dairy products).	No known symptoms due to cobalt deficiency.

Minerals

Copper: Component of enzymes that function in energy production, amino acid metabolism, and iron metabolism. Necessary for making hemoglobin.	RDA not established; estimated need is about 2 mg per day.	Liver, oysters, other seafood, and green vegetables are good sources. Dairy foods, meats, cereals are relatively poor sources.	Not seen in human adults. In infants and children with poor diets, copper deficiency may contribute to anemia and poor bone development.
Fluorine: Necessary in teeth to provide maximum protection against decay. May contribute to maintenance of bone structure.	RDA not established; recommend addition to drinking water to provide about 1 mg per quart.	Most foods contain only small amounts. Seafoods are fair sources. Tea and small fish eaten with bones (sardines) are good sources.	In infants and children deficiency may have adverse effects on bone structure and strength.
Iodine: Component of hormones produced by the thyroid gland. These regulate energy metabolism.	RDA: men: 130 µg; women: 100 µg	Iodized salt and seafoods are excellent sources. Bread made by continuous-mix process has high content.	Deficiency affects function of thyroid gland and produces goiter. Severe deficiency causes impairment of physical and mental development.
Iron: Component of hemoglobin, which transports oxygen from the lungs to the cells of the body. Also part of many enzymes involved in energy production.	RDA: men: 10 mg; women: 18 mg	Red meats and cereal foods enriched with iron are best sources. Liver is especially high in iron.	Deficiency causes anemia or low hemoglobin concentrations. Especially prevalent in infants and pregnant women.

Minerals

MINERALS (CONTINUED)

Mineral	RDA or Estimated Requirement for Adults	Food Sources	Deficiency
Manganese: Needed for normal bone structure, reproduction, and nerve function. Component of enzymes.	RDA not established; intakes of 2.5 to 7 mg per day meet requirements.	Nuts and whole-grain cereals are best sources. Tea is high in manganese. Fruits and vegetables are good sources; meats and seafood are not.	No evidence of manganese deficiency in humans.
Molybdenum: Component of several enzymes; possibly involved in iron metabolism.	RDA not established; tentative estimate is about 150 µg per day.	Content in foods varies widely. Good sources include legumes, whole-grain cereal products, milk, leafy vegetables, and organ meats.	No evidence of molybdenum deficiency in humans.
Nickel: Apparently functions in liver oxidation reactions in rats and chicks.	Believed but not proved essential for humans.	More research is necessary to determine food content.	No evidence of deficiency in humans.

Minerals

Selenium: Component of enzyme involved in maintaining integrity of cell membranes; may be important for protein synthesis; has antioxidant properties; may protect against toxicity of heavy metals (e.g., mercury).

RDA not established; actual human need not known.

Seafoods and meat have relatively high amounts. Fruits and vegetables are poor sources. Selenium content of foods varies widely depending on the soil in which they are grown.

No identification in humans of any symptoms resulting from selenium deficiency.

Silicon: Important for normal development of bones and connective tissues in rats and chicks.

Believed but not proved essential for humans.

No information available. (Silicon is one of the elements in sand and glass.)

No evidence of deficiency in humans.

Tin: Appears necessary for normal growth and tooth development in rats.

Not proved essential for humans; assume daily intake of 3.5 mg meets any nutritional requirement.

No solid information available; may be incorporated into foods from tinfoil and cans, although practice of lacquering cans reduces tin content of canned foods.

No evidence of deficiency in humans.

Vanadium: Promotes normal growth and reproductive ability in chicks and rats.

Probably essential for humans, but requirement is not known.

Little available information; food content appears to vary widely.

No evidence of deficiency in humans.

Minerals

MINERALS (CONTINUED)

Mineral	RDA or Estimated Requirement for Adults	Food Sources	Deficiency
Zinc: Constituent of many important enzymes; necessary for normal growth and sexual maturity; appears to be involved in wound healing.	RDA: 15 mg	Seafoods, especially oysters, are rich in zinc. Red meats and some cheeses are good sources. Whole-grain foods, nuts, dried peas and beans furnish good amounts.	Conditions in humans related to zinc deficiency include: growth failure, sexual immaturity, impaired wound healing, and reduced taste sensation.

Compiled from:
Food and Nutrition Board — National Research Council: *Recommended Dietary Allowances*, Eighth edition. National Academy of Sciences, Washington, D.C., 1974.
Trace Elements in Human Nutrition, Report of a WHO Expert Committee. World Health Organization Technical Report Series No. 532, Geneva, Switzerland, 1973.
Chaney, M; Ross, M; Witschi, J: *Nutrition*, Ninth edition, Houghton Mifflin Co., Boston, 1979.

Vitamin Supplement Profiles

CONSUMER GUIDE® magazine does not recommend the use of single vitamin or vitamin-mineral supplements by persons who are in good health and who eat a balanced diet. The only one who can really determine whether or not you need a supplementary source of vitamins and minerals is your physician after a careful evaluation of your diet and eating habits.

In this chapter nearly 70 of the vitamin and vitamin-mineral drug products most commonly used in this country are profiled. In each profile you will find the product name, the manufacturer, each one's dosage from (e.g., capsule,

> *NOTE: Vitamin supplement formulations are accurate at time of printing, but subject to change without notice. The spelling "thiamine" is used rather than the more common spelling "thiamin" because manufacturers use the former spelling on their product labels.*

Vitamin Supplement Profiles

tablet) and the nutrients contained and their amounts. Where appropriate, possible side effects and comments pertaining to the product are listed. Some drugs are counterproductive in people with certain conditions. These conditions are outlined under "Contraindications." If you have a condition listed in this category, consult your physician before taking the product.

Although it is our contention throughout this book that eating with an eye on the RDA will provide you with all the nutrients you need from your daily diet, health circumstances change, and there may be occasion for you to take a vitamin supplement. Before purchasing any of the following products, however, a visit to your physician will determine if you really need a supplement and, if so, how much. Also, read the chapter entitled Vitamin Supplements for a full understanding of these products.

Abdec Baby Drops multivitamin

Manufacturer: Parke, Davis & Company
Dosage Form: Liquid
Ingredients: Content per 0.6 ml: vitamin A palmitate, 5000 IU; vitamin D, 400 IU; ascorbic acid (vitamin C), 50 mg; thiamine hydrochloride (vitamin B_1), 1.0 mg; riboflavin (vitamin B_2), 1.2 mg; niacinamide, 10 mg; pyridoxine hydrochloride, 1.0 mg; sodium pantothenate, 5.0 mg
Comments: Abdec Baby Drops multivitamin contains ingredients which accumulate and are stored in the body. The recommended dose should not be exceeded for long periods (several weeks to months) except by physician's orders.

Abdec Baby Drops multivitamin will taste better chilled although refrigeration is not required for its stability.

Abdec Baby Drops multivitamin contains vitamin A in amounts (per liquid measure) greater than 100 percent of the U.S. RDA for "Infants from birth to 1 year" and "Children under 4 years." This amount is not toxic, however.

Vitamin Supplement Profiles

Abdec Kapseals multivitamin

Manufacturer: Parke, Davis & Company
Dosage Form: Capsule
Ingredients: vitamin A palmitate, 10,000 IU; vitamin D, 400 IU; vitamin E, 5 IU; ascorbic acid (vitamin C), 75 mg; thiamine mononitrate (vitamin B_1), 5.0 mg; riboflavin (vitamin B_2), 3.0 mg; niacinamide, 25 mg; pyridoxine hydrochloride (vitamin B_6), 1.5 mg; cyanocobalamin (vitamin B_{12}), 2.0 µg; pantothenic acid, 10 mg
Comments: Abdec Kapseals multivitamin contains ingredients which accumulate and are stored in the body. The recommended dose should not be exceeded for long periods (several weeks to months) except by physician's orders.

Abdec Kapseals multivitamin contains one or more vitamin or mineral in amounts (per capsule) greater than 100 percent of the U.S. RDA. Vitamins or minerals are not present in toxic amounts, however.

Abdol with Minerals multivitamin

Manufacturer: Parke, Davis & Company
Dosage Form: Capsule
Ingredients: vitamin A palmitate, 5000 IU; vitamin D, 400 IU; ascorbic acid (vitamin C), 50 mg; thiamine mononitrate, 2.5 mg; riboflavin (vitamin B_2), 2.5 mg; niacinamide, 20 mg; pyridoxine hydrochloride (vitamin B_6), 0.5 mg; cyanocobalamin (vitamin B_{12}), 1.0 µg; folic acid, 100 µg; calcium pantothenate, 2.5 mg; ferrous sulfate, 15 mg; calcium, 44.0 mg; phosphorus, 34.0 mg; magnesium, 1.0 mg; potassium sulfate, 5.0 mg; manganese sulfate, 1.0 mg; zinc sulfate, 0.5 mg. Abdol with Minerals multivitamin also contains trace quantities of iodine and copper.
Comments: Accidental iron poisoning is common in children; so be sure to keep Abdol with Minerals multivitamin safely out of their reach.

Vitamin Supplement Profiles

Abdol with Minerals multivitamin contains ingredients which accumulate and are stored in the body. The recommended dose should not be exceeded for long periods (several weeks to months) except by physician's orders.

The iron in Abdol with Minerals multivitamin interacts with oral tetracycline hydrochloride and reduces the absorption of the antibiotic. Consult your pharmacist or physician.

Abdol with Minerals multivitamin contains one or more vitamin or mineral in amounts (per capsule) greater than 100 percent of the U.S. RDA. Vitamins or minerals are not present in toxic amounts, however.

Adabee multivitamin

Manufacturer: A. H. Robins Company
Dosage Form: Tablet
Ingredients: vitamin A, 10,000 IU; sodium ascorbate (vitamin C), 250 mg; thiamine mononitrate, 15 mg; riboflavin (vitamin B_2), 10 mg; niacinamide, 50 mg; pyridoxine hydrochloride (vitamin B_6), 5 mg
Comments: Adabee multivitamin contains ingredients which accumulate and are stored in the body. The recommended dose should not be exceeded for long periods (several weeks to months) except by physician's orders.

Adabee multivitamin contains vitamin B_6 which may interact with levodopa (L-Dopa).

If two or more tablets are taken daily, Adabee multivitamin may interfere with the results of urine tests. Tell your physician and pharmacist you are taking this product.

Adabee multivitamin contains one or more vitamin or mineral in amounts (per tablet) greater than 100 percent of the U.S. RDA. Vitamins or minerals are not present in toxic amounts, however.

Vitamin Supplement Profiles

Adabee with Minerals multivitamin

Manufacturer: A. H. Robins Company
Dosage Form: Tablet
Ingredients: vitamin A, 10,000 IU; sodium ascorbate (vitamin C), 250 mg; thiamine mononitrate (vitamin B_1), 15 mg; riboflavin (vitamin B_2), 10 mg; niacinamide, 50 mg; pyridoxine hydrochloride (vitamin B_6), 5 mg; iron, 15 mg; calcium, 103 mg; phosphorus, 80 mg
Comments: Accidental iron poisoning is common in children; so be sure to keep Adabee with Minerals multivitamin safely out of their reach.

Adabee with Minerals multivitamin contains ingredients which accumulate and are stored in the body. The recommended dose should not be exceeded for long periods (several weeks to months) except by physician's orders.

Adabee with Minerals multivitamin contains vitamin B_6 which may interact with levodopa (L-Dopa).

The iron in Adabee with Minerals multivitamin interacts with oral tetracycline hydrochloride and reduces the absorption of the antibiotic. Consult your pharmacist or physician.

If two or more tablets are taken daily, Adabee with Minerals multivitamin may interfere with the results of urine tests. Tell your physician and pharmacist you are taking this product.

Adabee with Minerals multivitamin contains one or more vitamin or mineral in amounts (per tablet) greater than 100 percent of the U.S. RDA. Vitamins or minerals are not present in toxic amounts, however.

Allbee multivitamin

Manufacturer: A. H. Robins Company
Dosage Form: Capsule
Ingredients: ascorbic acid (vitamin C), 300 mg; thiamine mononitrate (vitamin B_1), 15 mg; riboflavin (vitamin B_2),

Vitamin Supplement Profiles

10.2 mg; niacinamide, 50 mg; pyridoxine hydrochloride (vitamin B_6), 5 mg; calcium pantothenate, 10 mg

Comments: Allbee multivitamin contains vitamin B_6 which may interact with levodopa (L-Dopa).

If two or more capsules are taken daily, Allbee multivitamin may interfere with the results of urine tests. Tell your physician and pharmacist you are taking this product.

Allbee multivitamin contains one or more vitamin or mineral in amounts (per capsule) greater than 100 percent of the U.S. RDA. Vitamins or minerals are not present in toxic amounts, however.

Chocks multivitamin (regular and Bugs Bunny)

Manufacturer: Miles Laboratories, Inc.
Dosage Form: Chewable tablet
Ingredients: vitamin A, 5000 IU; vitamin D, 400 IU; vitamin E, 15 IU; ascorbic acid (vitamin C), 60 mg; thiamine (vitamin B_1), 1.5 mg; riboflavin (vitamin B_2), 1.7 mg; niacin, 20 mg; pyridoxine hydrochloride (vitamin B_6), 2 mg; cyanocobalamin (vitamin B_{12}), 6 µg; folic acid 400 µg

Comments: Chocks multivitamin (regular and Bugs Bunny) contains ingredients which accumulate and are stored in the body. The recommended dose should not be exceeded for long periods (several weeks to months) except by physician's orders.

Chewable tablets should never be referred to as "candy" or as "candy-flavored" vitamins. Your child may take you literally and swallow toxic amounts.

Chocks Plus Iron multivitamin (regular and Bugs Bunny Plus Iron)

Manufacturer: Miles Laboratories, Inc.
Dosage Form: Chewable tablet
Ingredients: vitamin A, 5000 IU; vitamin D, 400 IU; vitamin

Vitamin Supplement Profiles

E, 15 IU; ascorbic acid (vitamin C), 60 mg; thiamine (vitamin B_1), 1.5 mg; riboflavin (vitamin B_2), 1.7 mg; niacin, 20 mg; pyridoxine hydrochloride (vitamin B_6), 2 mg; cyanocobalamin (vitamin B_{12}), 6 µg; folic acid, 400 µg; iron, 15 mg

Comments: Accidental iron poisoning is common in children; so be sure to keep Chocks Plus Iron multivitamin (regular and Bugs Bunny Plus Iron) safely out of their reach.

Chocks Plus Iron multivitamin (regular and Bugs Bunny Plus Iron) contains ingredients which accumulate and are stored in the body. The recommended dose should not be exceeded for long periods (several weeks to months) except by physician's orders.

Chewable tablets should never be referred to as "candy" or as "candy-flavored" vitamins. Your child may take you literally and swallow toxic amounts.

The iron in Chocks Plus Iron multivitamin (regular and Bugs Bunny Plus Iron) interacts with oral tetracycline hydrochloride and reduces the absorption of the antibiotic. Consult your pharmacist or physician.

Cod Liver Oil Concentrate multivitamin

Manufacturer: Schering Corporation
Dosage Forms: Capsule; tablet
Ingredients: Capsule: vitamin A, 10,000 IU; vitamin D, 400 IU. Tablet: vitamin A, 4000 IU; vitamin D, 200 IU
Comments: Cod Liver Oil Concentrate multivitamin contains ingredients which accumulate and are stored in the body. The recommended dose should not be exceeded for long periods (several weeks to months) except by physician's orders.

The capsule form of Cod Liver Oil Concentrate multivitamin contains vitamin A in amounts (per capsule) greater than 100 percent of the U.S. RDA. This amount is not toxic, however.

Vitamin Supplement Profiles

Combex Kapseals with Vitamin C multivitamin

Manufacturer: Parke, Davis & Company
Dosage Form: Capsule
Ingredients: ascorbic acid (vitamin C), 50 mg; thiamine mononitrate (vitamin B_1), 10 mg; riboflavin (vitamin B_2), 10 mg; niacinamide, 10 mg; cyanocobalamin (vitamin B_{12}), 1 µg; panthenol, 6 mg; liver concentrate, 340 mg
Comments: Combex Kapseals with Vitamin C multivitamin contains ingredients which accumulate and are stored in the body. The recommended dose should not be exceeded for long periods (several weeks to months) except by physician's orders.

Combex Kapseals with Vitamin C multivitamin contains one or more vitamin or mineral in amounts (per capsule) greater than 100 percent of the U.S. RDA. Vitamins or minerals are not present in toxic amounts.

Dayalets multivitamin

Manufacturer: Abbott Laboratories
Dosage Form: Tablet
Ingredients: vitamin A, 5000 IU; vitamin D, 400 IU; vitamin E, 30 IU; ascorbic acid (vitamin C), 60 mg; thiamine hydrochloride (vitamin B_1), 1.5 mg; riboflavin (vitamin B_2), 1.7 mg; niacinamide, 20 mg; pyridoxine hydrochloride (vitamin B_6), 2 mg; cyanocobalamin (vitamin B_{12}), 6 µg; folic acid, 400 µg
Comments: Dayalets multivitamin contains ingredients which accumulate and are stored in the body. The recommended dose should not be exceeded for long periods (several weeks to months) except by physician's orders.

Dayalets plus Iron multivitamin

Manufacturer: Abbott Laboratories
Dosage Form: Tablet

Vitamin Supplement Profiles

Ingredients: vitamin A, 5000 IU; vitamin D, 400 IU; vitamin E, 30 IU; ascorbic acid (vitamin C), 60 mg; thiamine hydrochloride (vitamin B_1), 1.5 mg; riboflavin (vitamin B_2), 1.7 mg; niacinamide, 20 mg; pyridoxine hydrochloride (vitamin B_6), 2 mg; cyanocobalamin (vitamin B_{12}), 6 µg; folic acid, 400 µg; iron, 18 mg

Comments: Accidental iron poisoning is common in children; so be sure to keep Dayalets plus Iron multivitamin safely out of their reach.

Dayalets plus Iron multivitamin contains ingredients which accummulate and are stored in the body. The recommended dose should not be exceeded for long periods (several weeks to months) except by physician's orders.

The iron in Dayalets plus Iron multivitamin interacts with oral tetracycline hydrochloride and reduces the absorption of the antibiotic. Consult your pharmacist or physician.

Di-Cal D multivitamin

Manufacturer: Abbott Laboratories
Dosage Form: Capsule
Ingredients: vitamin D, 133 IU; calcium 116 mg; phosphorus, 90 mg
Comments: Di-Cal D multivitamin contains ingredients which accumulate and are stored in the body. The recommended dose should not be exceeded for long periods (several weeks to months) except by physician's orders.

Femiron iron supplement

Manufacturer: J.B. Williams Co., Inc.
Dosage Form: Tablet
Ingredients: ferrous fumarate, 63 mg
Comments: Accidental iron poisoning is common in children; so be sure to keep Femiron iron supplement

Vitamin Supplement Profiles

safely out of their reach.

The iron in Femiron iron supplement interacts with oral tetracycline hydrochloride and reduces the absorption of the antibiotic. Consult your pharmacist or physician.

Femiron iron supplement releases 20 mg of elemental iron per dose, which is slightly greater than 100 percent of the U.S. RDA. This amount is not toxic, however.

Femiron multivitamin

Manufacturer: J. B. Williams Co., Inc.
Dosage Form: Tablet
Ingredients: vitamin A, 5000 IU; vitamin D, 400 IU; ascorbic acid (vitamin C), 60 mg; thiamine (vitamin B_1), 1.5 mg; riboflavin (vitamin B_2), 1.7 mg; niacinamide, 20 mg; pyridoxine hydrochloride (vitamin B_6), 2 mg; cyanocobalamin (vitamin B_{12}), 5 µg; folic acid, 100 µg; calcium pantothenate, 10 mg; ferrous fumarate, 63 mg
Comments: Accidental iron poisoning is common in children; so be sure to keep Femiron multivitamin safely out of their reach.

Femiron multivitamin contains ingredients which accumulate and are stored in the body. The recommended dose should not be exceeded for long periods (several weeks to months) except by physician's orders.

The iron in Femiron multivitamin interacts with oral tetracycline hydrochloride and reduces the absorption of the antibiotic. Consult your pharmacist or physician.

Femiron multivitamin releases 20 mg of elemental iron per dose, which is slightly greater than 100 percent of the U.S. RDA. This amount is not toxic, however.

Feosol iron supplement

Manufacturer: Smith Kline & French Laboratories
Dosage Forms: Spansule capsule; tablet
Ingredients: Spansule capsule: ferrous sulfate, 167 mg.

Vitamin Supplement Profiles

Tablet: ferrous sulfate, 200 mg
Comments: Accidental iron poisoning is common in children; so be sure to keep Feosol iron supplement safely out of their reach.

The iron in Feosol iron supplement interacts with oral tetracycline hydrochloride and reduces the absorption of the antibiotic. Consult your pharmacist or physician.

Fergon iron supplement

Manufacturer: Breon Laboratories, Inc.
Dosage Forms: Capsule; tablet
Ingredients: Capsule: ferrous gluconate, 435 mg. Tablet: ferrous sulfate, 320 mg
Side Effects: Stomach pain, nausea, diarrhea, constipation
Contraindications: Fergon iron supplement is contraindicated for persons with active peptic ulcer or ulcerative colitis.
Comments: Fergon iron supplement contains iron which may cause nausea, stomach pain, diarrhea, or constipation. These symptoms usually disappear or become less severe after two to three days. Take Fergon iron supplement with food or milk to help minimize these effects. If they persist, ask your pharmacist to recommend another product.

Stools may be dark; this is a normal consequence of iron therapy.

Accidental iron poisoning is common in children; so be sure to keep Fergon iron supplement safely out of their reach.

The iron in Fergon iron supplement interacts with oral tetracycline hydrochloride and reduces the absorption of the antibiotic. Consult your pharmacist or physician.

Fergon iron supplement contains iron in amounts (per capsule; tablet) greater than 100 percent of the U.S. RDA. This amount is not toxic, however.

Vitamin Supplement Profiles

Fer-In-Sol iron supplement

Manufacturer: Mead Johnson Nutritional Division
Dosage Forms: Drop; syrup; capsule
Ingredients: Content per 0.6 ml (drop): ferrous sulfate, 75 mg. Content per 5 ml (syrup): ferrous sulfate, 150 mg. Capsule: ferrous sulfate, 190 mg
Comments: Accidental iron poisoning is common in children; so be sure to keep Fer-In-Sol iron supplement safely out of their reach.

The iron in Fer-In-Sol iron supplement interacts with oral tetracycline hydrochloride and reduces the absorption of the antibiotic. Consult your pharmacist or physician.

Fer-In-Sol iron supplement contains iron in amounts (per liquid measure; capsule) greater than 100 percent of the U.S. RDA. This amount is not toxic, however.

Flintstones multivitamin

Manufacturer: Miles Laboratories, Inc.
Dosage Form: Chewable tablet
Ingredients: vitamin A, 2500 IU; vitamin D, 400 IU; vitamin E, 15 IU; ascorbic acid (vitamin C), 60 mg; thiamine (vitamin B_1), 1.05 mg; riboflavin (vitamin B_2), 1.2 mg; niacin, 13.5 mg; pyridoxine hydrochloride (vitamin B_6), 1.05 mg; cyanocobalamin (vitamin B_{12}), 4.5 μg; folic acid, 300 μg
Comments: Flintstones multivitamin contains ingredients which accumulate and are stored in the body. The recommended dose should not be exceeded for long periods (several weeks to months) except by physician's orders.

Chewable tablets should never be referred to as "candy" or as "candy-flavored" vitamins. Your child may take you literally and swallow toxic amounts.

Vitamin Supplement Profiles

Flintstones Plus Iron multivitamin

Manufacturer: Miles Laboratories, Inc.
Dosage Form: Chewable tablet
Ingredients: vitamin A, 2500 IU; vitamin D, 400 IU; vitamin E, 15 IU; ascorbic acid (vitamin C), 60 mg; thiamine (vitamin B_1), 1.05 mg; riboflavin (vitamin B_2), 1.2 mg; niacin, 13.5 mg; pyridoxine hydrochloride (vitamin B_6), 1.05 mg; cyanocobalamin (vitamin B_{12}), 4.5 µg; folic acid, 0.3 mg; iron, 15 mg
Comments: Accidental iron poisoning is common in children; so be sure to keep Flintstones Plus Iron multivitamin safely out of their reach.

Chewable tablets should never be referred to as "candy" or as "candy-flavored" vitamins. Your child may take you literally and swallow toxic amounts.

The iron in Flintstones Plus Iron multivitamin interacts with oral tetracycline hydrochloride and reduces the absorption of the antibiotic. Consult your pharmacist or physician.

Geritol Junior multivitamin (liquid)

Manufacturer: J. B. Williams Co., Inc.
Dosage Form: Liquid
Ingredients: Content per 5 ml: vitamin A palmitate, 8000 IU; vitamin D, 400 IU; thiamine (vitamin B_1), 5 mg; riboflavin (vitamin B_2), 5 mg; niacinamide, 100 mg; pyridoxine hydrochloride (vitamin B_6), 1 mg; cyanocobalamin (vitamin B_{12}), 3 µg; panthenol, 4 mg; iron ammonium citrate, 100 mg
Comments: Geritol Junior multivitamin (liquid) will taste better chilled, although refrigeration is not required for its stability.

Accidental iron poisoning is common in children; so be sure to keep Geritol Junior multivitamin (liquid) safely out of their reach.

Geritol Junior multivitamin (liquid) contains ingre-

Vitamin Supplement Profiles

dients which accumulate and are stored in the body. The recommended dose should not be exceeded for long periods (several weeks to months) except by physician's orders.

The form of iron in Geritol Junior multivitamin (liquid) is not absorbed into the bloodstream as well as that in other products. If you are taking this product expressly for the iron content, ask your pharmacist to recommend another product.

The iron in Geritol Junior multivitamin (liquid) interacts with oral tetracycline hydrochloride and reduces the absorption of the antibiotic. Consult your pharmacist or physician.

Geritol Junior multivitamin (liquid) contains one or more vitamin or mineral in amounts (per liquid measure) greater than 100 percent of the U.S. RDA. Vitamins or minerals are not present in toxic amounts, however.

Geritol Junior multivitamin (tablet)

Manufacturer: J. B. Williams Co., Inc.
Dosage Form: Tablet
Ingredients: vitamin A, 5000 IU; vitamin D, 100 IU; ascorbic acid (vitamin C), 30 mg; thiamine (vitamin B_1), 2.5 mg; riboflavin (vitamin B_2), 2.5 mg; niacinamide, 20 mg; pyridoxine hydrochloride (vitamin B_6), 1 mg; cyanocobalamin (vitamin B_{12}), 2.5 μg; calcium pantothenate, 2 mg; ferrous sulfate, 25 mg
Comments: Accidental iron poisoning is common in children; so be sure to keep Geritol Junior multivitamin (tablet) safely out of their reach.

Geritol Junior multivitamin (tablet) contains ingredients which accumulate and are stored in the body. The recommended dose should not be exceeded for long periods (several weeks to months) except by physician's orders.

The iron in Geritol Junior multivitamin (tablet) interacts with oral tetracycline hydrochloride and reduces the

Vitamin Supplement Profiles

absorption of the antibiotic. Consult your pharmacist or physician.

Geritol Junior multivitamin (tablet) contains one or more vitamin or mineral in amounts (per tablet) greater than 100 percent of the U.S. RDA. Vitamins or minerals are not present in toxic amounts, however.

Geritol multivitamin (liquid)

Manufacturer: J.B. Williams Co., Inc.
Dosage Form: Liquid
Ingredients: Content per fluid ounce: thiamine (vitamin B_1), 5 mg; riboflavin (vitamin B_2), 5 mg; niacinamide, 100 mg; pyridoxine hydrochloride (vitamin B_6), 1 mg; cyanocobalamin (vitamin B_{12}), 3 µg; panthenol, 4 mg; iron ammonium citrate, 100 mg; methionine, 75 mg; choline bitartrate, 100 mg
Comments: The need for dietary supplements of methionine and choline bitartrate has not been demonstrated.

Geritol multivitamin (liquid) will taste better chilled, although refrigeration is not required for its stability.

Accidental iron poisoning is common in children; so be sure to keep Geritol multivitamin (liquid) safely out of their reach.

The form of iron in Geritol multivitamin (liquid) is not absorbed into the bloodstream as well as that in other products. If you are taking this product expressly for the iron content, ask your pharmacist to recommend another product.

The iron in Geritol multivitamin (liquid) interacts with oral tetracycline hydrochloride and reduces the absorption of the antibiotic. Consult your pharmacist or physician.

Geritol multivitamin (liquid) contains one or more vitamin or mineral in amounts (per liquid measure) greater than 100 percent of the U.S. RDA. Vitamins or minerals are not present in toxic amounts, however.

Vitamin Supplement Profiles

Geritol multivitamin (tablet)

Manufacturer: J. B. Williams Co., Inc.
Dosage Form: Tablet
Ingredients: ascorbic acid (vitamin C), 75 mg; thiamine (vitamin B_1), 5 mg; riboflavin (vitamin B_2), 5 mg; niacinamide, 30 mg; pyridoxine hydrochloride (vitamin B_6), 0.5 mg; cyanocobalamin (vitamin B_{12}), 3 µg; calcium pantothenate, 2 mg; ferrous sulfate, 50 mg
Comments: Accidental iron poisoning is common in children; so be sure to keep Geritol multivitamin (tablet) safely out of their reach.

The iron in Geritol multivitamin (tablet) interacts with oral tetracycline hydrochloride and reduces the absorption of the antibiotic. Consult your pharmacist or physician.

Geritol multivitamin (tablet) contains one or more vitamin or mineral in amounts (per tablet) greater than 100 percent of the U.S. RDA. Vitamins or minerals are not present in toxic amounts, however.

Gevrabon multivitamin

Manufacturer: Lederle Laboratories
Dosage Form: Liquid
Ingredients: Content per 30 ml: thiamine (vitamin B_1), 5 mg; riboflavin (vitamin B_2), 5 mg; niacinamide, 50 mg; pyridoxine hydrochloride (vitamin B_6), 1 mg; cyanocobalamin (vitamin B_{12}), 1 µg; pantothenic acid, 10 mg; iron, 15 mg; magnesium, 2 mg; iodine, 100 µg; inositol, 100 mg; choline, 100 mg; manganese, 2 mg; zinc, 2 mg; phosphate sodium, 2.5 mg
Comments: The need for supplementary choline and inositol in humans has not been demonstrated.

Accidental iron poisoning is common in children; so be sure to keep Gevrabon multivitamin safely out of their reach.

Gevrabon multivitamin will taste better chilled,

Vitamin Supplement Profiles

although refrigeration is not required for its stability.

Gevrabon multivitamin contains one or more vitamin or mineral in amounts (per liquid measure) greater than 100 percent of the U.S. RDA. Vitamins or minerals are not present in toxic amounts, however.

Iberet-500 multivitamin (oral solution)

Manufacturer: Abbott Laboratories
Dosage Form: Liquid
Ingredients: Content per 5 ml: ascorbic acid (vitamin C), 125 mg; thiamine hydrochloride (vitamin B_1), 1.5 mg; riboflavin (vitamin B_2), 1.5 mg; niacinamide, 7.5 mg; pyridoxine hydochloride (vitamin B_6), 1.25 mg; cyanocobalamin (vitamin B_{12}), 6.25 μg; panthenol, 2.5 mg; iron, 26.2 mg
Comments: Accidental iron poisoning is common in children; so be sure to keep Iberet-500 multivitamin (oral solution) safely out of their reach.

Iberet-500 multivitamin (oral solution) will taste better chilled, although refrigeration is not required for its stability.

The iron in Iberet-500 multivitamin (oral solution) interacts with oral tetracycline hydrochloride and reduces the absorption of the antibiotic. Consult your pharmacist or physician.

Iberet-500 multivitamin (oral solution) contains one or more vitamin or mineral in amounts (per liquid measure) greater than 100 percent of the U.S. RDA. Vitamins or minerals are not present in toxic amounts, however.

Iberet-500 multivitamin (tablet)

Manufacturer: Abbott Laboratories
Dosage Form: Tablet
Ingredients: sodium ascorbate (vitamin C), 500 mg; thiamine hydrochloride (vitamin B_1), 6 mg; riboflavin (vitamin B_2), 6 mg; niacinamide, 30 mg; pyridoxine

Vitamin Supplement Profiles

hydrochloride (vitamin B_6), 5 mg; cyanocobalamin (vitamin B_{12}), 25 µg; calcium pantothenate, 10 mg; iron, 105 mg

Side Effects: Stomach pain, nausea, diarrhea, constipation

Contraindications: Iberet-500 multivitamin (tablet) is contraindicated for persons with active peptic ulcer or ulcerative colitis.

Comments: Iberet-500 multivitamin (tablet) contains iron which may cause nausea, stomach pain, diarrhea, or constipation. These symptoms usually disappear or become less severe after two to three days. Take Iberet-500 multivitamin (tablet) with food or milk to help minimize these effects. If they persist, ask your pharmacist to recommend another product.

Accidental iron poisoning is common in children; so be sure to keep Iberet-500 multivitamin (tablet) safely out of their reach.

Iberet-500 multivitamin (tablet) contains vitamin B_6 which may interact with levodopa (L-Dopa).

The iron in Iberet-500 multivitamin (tablet) interacts with oral tetracycline hydrochloride and reduces the absorption of the antibiotic. Consult your pharmacist or physician.

Iberet-500 multivitamin (tablet) may interfere with the results of urine tests. Tell your physician and pharmacist you are taking this product.

Iberet-500 multivitamin (tablet) contains one or more vitamin or mineral in amounts (per tablet) greater than 100 percent of the U.S. RDA. Vitamins or minerals are not present in toxic amounts, however.

Iberet multivitamin (oral solution)

Manufacturer: Abbott Laboratories
Dosage Form: Liquid
Ingredients: Content per 5 ml: ascorbic acid (vitamin C), 37.5 mg; thiamine hydrochloride (vitamin B_1), 1.5 mg;

Vitamin Supplement Profiles

riboflavin (vitamin B_2), 1.5 mg; niacinamide, 7.5 mg; pyridoxine hydrochloride (vitamin B_6), 1.25 mg; cyanocobalamin (vitamin B_{12}), 6.25 µg; panthenol, 2.5 mg; iron, 26 mg

Comments: Accidental iron poisoning is common in children; so be sure to keep Iberet multivitamin (oral solution) safely out of their reach.

Iberet multivitamin (oral solution) will taste better chilled, although refrigeration is not required for its stability.

The iron in Iberet multivitamin (oral solution) interacts with oral tetracycline hydrochloride and reduces the absorption of the antibiotic. Consult your pharmacist or physician.

Iberet multivitamin (oral solution) contains one or more vitamin or mineral in amounts (per liquid measure) greater than 100 percent of the U.S. RDA. Vitamins or minerals are not present in toxic amounts, however.

Iberet multivitamin (tablet)

Manufacturer: Abbott Laboratories
Dosage Form: Tablet
Ingredients: sodium ascorbate (vitamin C), 150 mg; thiamine hydrochloride (vitamin B_1), 6 mg; riboflavin (vitamin B_2), 6 mg; niacinamide, 30 mg; pyridoxine hydrochloride (vitamin B_6), 5 mg; cyanocobalamin (vitamin B_{12}), 25 µg; calcium pantothenate, 10 mg; iron, 105 mg

Comments: Accidental iron poisoning is common in children; so be sure to keep Iberet multivitamin (tablet) safely out of their reach.

Iberet multivitamin (tablet) contains vitamin B_6 which may interact with levodopa (L-Dopa).

The iron in Iberet multivitamin (tablet) interacts with oral tetracycline hydrochloride and reduces the absorption of the antibiotic. Consult your pharmacist or physician.

Vitamin Supplement Profiles

Iberet multivitamin (tablet) contains one or more vitamin or mineral in amounts (per tablet) greater than 100 percent of the U.S. RDA. Vitamins or minerals are not present in toxic amounts, however.

Iberol multivitamin

Manufacturer: Abbott Laboratories
Dosage Form: Tablet
Ingredients: sodium ascorbate (vitamin C), 75 mg; thiamine mononitrate (vitamin B_1), 3 mg; riboflavin (vitamin B_2), 3 mg; niacinamide, 15 mg; pyridoxine hydrochloride (vitamin B_6), 1.5 mg; cyanocobalamin (vitamin B_{12}), 12.5 µg; calcium pantothenate, 3 mg; iron, 105 mg
Side Effects: Stomach pain, nausea, diarrhea, constipation
Contraindications: Iberol multivitamin is contraindicated for persons with active peptic ulcer or ulcerative colitis.
Comments: Iberol multivitamin contains iron which may cause nausea, stomach pain, diarrhea, or constipation. These symptoms usually disappear or become less severe after two to three days. Take Iberol multivitamin with food or milk to help minimize these effects. If they persist, ask your pharmacist to recommend another product.

Accidental iron poisoning is common in children; so be sure to keep Iberol multivitamin safely out of their reach.

The iron in Iberol multivitamin interacts with oral tetracycline hydrochloride and reduces the absorption of the antibiotic. Consult your pharmacist or physician.

Iberol multivitamin contains one or more vitamin or mineral in amounts (per tablet) greater than 100 percent of the U.S. RDA. Vitamins or minerals are not present in toxic amounts, however.

Vitamin Supplement Profiles

Incremin with Iron multivitamin

Manufacturer: Lederle Laboratories
Dosage Form: Syrup
Ingredients: Content per 5 ml: thiamine hydrochloride (vitamin B_1), 10 mg; pyridoxine hydrochloride (vitamin B_6), 5 mg; cyanocobalamin (vitamin B_{12}), 25 µg; iron pyrophosphate, 30 mg; sorbitol, 3.5 g; lysine monohydrochloride, 300 mg
Comments: Sorbitol and lysine monohydrochloride are not vitamins.

Accidental iron poisoning is common in children; so be sure to keep Incremin with Iron multivitamin safely out of their reach.

The form of iron in Incremin with Iron multivitamin is not absorbed into the bloodstream as well as other products. If you are taking this product expressly for the iron content, ask your pharmacist to recommend another product.

Incremin with Iron multivitamin contains vitamin B_6 which may interact with levodopa (L-Dopa).

Incremin with Iron multivitamin will taste better chilled, although refrigeration is not required for its stability.

The iron in Incremin with Iron multivitamin interacts with oral tetracycline hydrochloride and reduces the absorption of the antibiotic. Consult your pharmacist or physician.

Incremin with Iron multivitamin contains one or more vitamin or mineral in amounts (per liquid measure) greater than 100 percent of the U.S. RDA. Vitamins or minerals are not present in toxic amounts, however.

Ironized Yeast iron supplement

Manufacturer: Glenbrook Laboratories
Dosage Form: Tablet
Ingredients: ferrous sulfate, 56.88 mg; yeast, 384 mg; thiamine (vitamin B_1), 0.37 mg

Vitamin Supplement Profiles

Comments: Accidental iron poisoning is common in children; so be sure to keep Ironized Yeast iron supplement safely out of their reach.

The iron in Ironized Yeast iron supplement interacts with oral tetracycline hydrochloride and reduces the absorption of the antibiotic. Consult your pharmacist or physician.

Livitamin multivitamin (capsule)

Manufacturer: Beecham Laboratories
Dosage Form: Capsule
Ingredients: ascorbic acid (vitamin C), 100 mg; thiamine mononitrate (vitamin B_1), 3 mg; riboflavin (vitamin B_2), 3 mg; niacinamide, 10 mg; pyridoxine hydrochloride (vitamin B_6), 3 mg; cyanocobalamin (vitamin B_{12}), 5 µg; calcium pantothenate, 2 mg; iron, 33 mg; desiccated liver, 150 mg; copper, 0.66 mg
Comments: Accidental iron poisoning is common in children; so be sure to keep Livitamin multivitamin (capsule) safely out of their reach.

The iron in Livitamin multivitamin (capsule) interacts with oral tetracycline hydrochloride and reduces the absorption of the antibiotic. Consult your pharmacist or physician.

Livitamin multivitamin (capsule) contains vitamin B_6 which may interact with levodopa (L-Dopa). This interaction occurs only if two to three doses of Livitamin multivitamin (capsule) are taken each day.

Livitamin multivitamin (capsule) contains one or more vitamin or mineral in amounts (per capsule) greater than 100 percent of the U.S. RDA. Vitamins or minerals are not present in toxic amounts, however.

Livitamin multivitamin (chewable tablet)

Manufacturer: Beecham Laboratories
Dosage Form: Chewable tablet

Vitamin Supplement Profiles

Ingredients: ascorbic acid (vitamin C), 100 mg; thiamine mononitrate (vitamin B_1), 3 mg; riboflavin (vitamin B_2), 3 mg; niacinamide, 10 mg; pyridoxine hydrochloride (vitamin B_6), 3 mg; cyanocobalamin (vitamin B_{12}), 5 µg; calcium pantothenate, 2 mg; iron, 16.4 mg; copper, 0.33 mg

Comments: Accidental iron poisoning is common in children; so be sure to keep Livitamin multivitamin (chewable tablet) safely out of their reach.

Chewable tablets should never be referred to as "candy" or as "candy-flavored" vitamins. Your child may take you literally and swallow toxic amounts.

The iron in Livitamin multivitamin (chewable tablet) interacts with oral tetracycline hydrochloride and reduces the absorption of the antibiotic. Consult your pharmacist or physician.

Livitamin multivitamin (chewable tablet) contains vitamin B_6 which may interact with levodopa (L-Dopa). This interaction occurs only if two to three doses of Livitamin multivitamin (chewable tablet) are taken each day.

Livitamin multivitamin (chewable tablet) contains one or more vitamin or mineral in amounts (per tablet) greater than 100 percent of the U.S. RDA. Vitamins or minerals are not present in toxic amounts, however.

Livitamin multivitamin (liquid)

Manufacturer: Beecham Laboratories
Dosage Form: Liquid
Ingredients: Content per 15 ml: thiamine hydrochloride (vitamin B_1), 3 mg; riboflavin (vitamin B_2), 3 mg; niacinamide, 10 mg; pyridoxine hydrochloride (vitamin B_6), 3 mg; cyanocobalamin (vitamin B_{12}), 5 µg; panthenol, 2 mg; iron, 35 mg; liver fraction 1, 500 mg; copper, 0.66 mg
Comments: Accidental iron poisoning is common in children; so be sure to keep Livitamin multivitamin (liquid) safely out of their reach.

Vitamin Supplement Profiles

Livitamin multivitamin (liquid) will taste better chilled, although refrigeration is not required for its stability.

The iron in Livitamin multivitamin (liquid) interacts with oral tetracycline hydrochloride and reduces the absorption of the antibiotic. Consult your pharmacist or physician.

Livitamin multivitamin (liquid) contains vitamin B_6 which may interact with levodopa (L-Dopa). This interaction occurs only if two to three doses of Livitamin multivitamin (liquid) are taken each day.

Livitamin multivitamin (liquid) contains one or more vitamin or mineral in amounts (per liquid measure) greater than 100 percent of the U.S. RDA. Vitamins or minerals are not present in toxic amounts, however.

Mol-Iron iron supplement

Manufacturer: Schering Corporation
Dosage Forms: Liquid; tablet
Ingredients: Content per 4 ml (liquid): ferrous sulfate, 195 mg. Tablet: ferrous sulfate, 390 mg
Side Effects: Tablet: stomach pain, nausea, diarrhea, constipation
Contraindications: The tablet form of Mol-Iron iron supplement is contraindicated for persons with active peptic ulcer or ulcerative colitis.
Comments: Because of the quantity of iron, the tablet form of Mol-Iron iron supplement may cause nausea, stomach pain, diarrhea, or constipation. These symptoms usually disappear or become less severe after two to three days. Take Mol-Iron iron supplement (tablet) with food or milk to help minimize these effects. If they persist, ask your pharmacist to recommend another product.

Stools may be dark when the tablet form is used; this is a normal consequence of iron therapy.

Accidental iron poisoning is common in children; so be

Vitamin Supplement Profiles

sure to keep Mol-Iron iron supplement safely out of their reach.

The iron in Mol-Iron iron supplement interacts with oral tetracycline hydrochloride and reduces the absorption of the antibiotic. Consult your pharmacist or physician.

Mol-Iron iron supplement contains iron in amounts (per liquid measure; tablet) greater than 100 percent of the U.S. RDA. Iron is not present in toxic amounts, however.

Monster Brand multivitamin

Manufacturer: Bristol-Myers Products
Dosage Form: Chewable tablet
Ingredients: vitamin A, 3500 IU; vitamin D, 400 IU; ascorbic acid (vitamin C), 40 mg; thiamine (vitamin B_1), 1.1 mg; riboflavin (vitamin B_2), 1.2 mg; niacin, 15 mg; pyridoxine hydrochloride (vitamin B_6), 1.2 mg; cyanocobalamin (vitamin B_{12}), 5 µg; folic acid, 100 µg; pantothenic acid, 5 mg
Comments: Monster Brand multivitamin contains ingredients which accumulate and are stored in the body. The recommended dose should not be exceeded for long periods (several weeks to months) except by physician's orders.

Chewable tablets should never be referred to as "candy" or as "candy-flavored" vitamins. Your child may take you literally and swallow toxic amounts.

Monster Brand multivitamin with iron

Manufacturer: Bristol-Myers Products
Dosage Form: Chewable tablet
Ingredients: vitamin A, 3500 IU; vitamin D, 400 IU; ascorbic acid (vitamin C), 40 mg; thiamine (vitamin B_1), 1.1 mg; riboflavin (vitamin B_2), 1.2 mg; niacinamide, 15

Vitamin Supplement Profiles

mg; pyridoxine hydrochloride (vitamin B$_6$), 1.2 mg; cyanocobalamin (vitamin B$_{12}$), 5 μg; folic acid, 100 μg; pantothenic acid, 5 mg; iron, 10 mg

Comments: Accidental iron poisoning is common in children; so be sure to keep Monster Brand multivitamin with iron safely out of their reach.

Monster Brand multivitamin with iron contains ingredients which accumulate and are stored in the body. The recommended dose should not be exceeded for long periods (several weeks to months) except by physician's orders.

Chewable tablets should never be referred to as "candy" or as "candy-flavored" vitamins. Your child may take you literally and swallow toxic amounts.

The iron in Monster Brand multivitamin with iron interacts with oral tetracycline hydrochloride and reduces the absorption of the antibiotic. Consult your pharmacist or physician.

Multicebrin multivitamin

Manufacturer: Eli Lilly and Company
Dosage Form: Capsule
Ingredients: vitamin A, 5000 IU; vitamin D, 500 IU; vitamin E, 2.5 IU; ascorbic acid (vitamin C), 56 mg; thiamine hydrochloride (vitamin B$_1$), 1.5 mg; riboflavin (vitamin B$_2$), 2 mg; niacin, 6 mg; pyridoxine hydrochloride (vitamin B$_6$), 1 mg; cyanocobalamin (vitamin B$_{12}$), 1.8 μg

Comments: Multicebrin multivitamin contains ingredients which accumulate and are stored in the body. The recommended dose should not be exceeded for long periods (several weeks to months) except by physician's orders.

Multicebrin multivitamin contains one or more vitamin or mineral in amounts (per capsule) greater than 100 percent of the U.S. RDA. Vitamins or minerals are not present in toxic amounts, however.

Vitamin Supplement Profiles

Myadec multivitamin

Manufacturer: Parke, Davis & Company
Dosage form: Tablet; capsule
Ingredients: vitamin A, 10,000 IU; vitamin D, 400 IU; vitamin E, 30 IU; ascorbic acid (vitamin C), 250 mg; thiamine mononitrate, 10 mg; riboflavin (vitamin B_2), 10 mg; niacinamide, 100 mg; pyridoxine hydrochloride (vitamin B_6), 5 mg; cyanocobalamin (vitamin B_{12}), 5 µg; iron, 20 mg; magnesium sulfate 25 mg; copper sulfate, 2 mg; zinc sulfate, 1.5 mg; manganese sulfate, 1 mg; potassium iodide, 150 µg
Comments: Accidental iron poisoning is common in children; so be sure to keep Myadec multivitamin safely out of their reach.

Myadec multivitamin contains ingredients which accumulate and are stored in the body. The recommended dose should not be exceeded for long periods (several weeks to months) except by physician's orders.

Myadec multivitamin contains vitamin B_6 which may interact with levodopa (L-Dopa).

The iron in Myadec multivitamin interacts with oral tetracycline hydrochloride and reduces the absorption of the antibiotic. Consult your pharmacist or physician.

If two or more tablets or capsules are taken daily, Myadec multivitamin may interfere with the results of urine tests. Tell your physician and pharmacist you are taking this product.

Myadec multivitamin contains one or more vitamin or mineral in amounts (per tablet; capsule) greater than 100 percent of the U.S. RDA. Vitamins or minerals are not present in toxic amounts, however.

One-A-Day multivitamin

Manufacturer: Miles Laboratories, Inc.
Dosage Form: Tablet
Ingredients: vitamin A, 5000 IU; vitamin D, 400 IU; vitamin

Vitamin Supplement Profiles

E, 15 IU; ascorbic acid (vitamin C), 60 mg; thiamine (vitamin B_1), 1.5 mg; riboflavin (vitamin B_2), 1.7 mg; niacin, 20 mg; pyridoxine hydrochloride (vitamin B_6), 2 mg; cyanocobalamin (vitamin B_{12}), 6 μg; folic acid, 400 μg

Comments: One-A-Day multivitamin contains ingredients which accumulate and are stored in the body. The recommended dose should not be exceeded for long periods (several weeks to months) except by physician's orders.

One-A-Day multivitamin plus iron

Manufacturer: Miles Laboratories, Inc.
Dosage Form: Capsule
Ingredients: vitamin A, 5000 IU; vitamin D, 400 IU; vitamin E, 15 IU; ascorbic acid (vitamin C), 60 mg; thiamine (vitamin B_1), 1.5 mg; riboflavin (vitamin B_2), 1.7 mg; niacin, 20 mg; pyridoxine hydrochloride (vitamin B_6), 2 mg; cyanocobalamin (vitamin B_{12}), 6 μg; folic acid, 400 μg; iron, 18 mg

Comments: Accidental iron poisoning is common in children; so be sure to keep One-A-Day multivitamin plus iron safely out of their reach.

One-A-Day multivitamin plus iron contains ingredients which accumulate and are stored in the body. The recommended dose should not be exceeded for long periods (several weeks to months) except by physician's orders.

The iron in One-A-Day multivitamin plus iron interacts with oral tetracycline hydrochloride and reduces the absorption of the antibiotic. Consult your pharmacist or physician.

One-A-Day multivitamin plus minerals

Manufacturer: Miles Laboratories, Inc.
Dosage Form: Capsule

Vitamin Supplement Profiles

Ingredients: zinc, 15 mg; copper, 2 mg; iodine, 150 µg; vitamin A, 5000 IU; vitamin D, 400 IU; vitamin E, 15 IU; ascorbic acid (vitamin C), 60 mg; thiamine (vitamin B_1), 1.5 mg; riboflavin (vitamin B2), 1.7 mg; niacin, 20 mg; pyridoxine hydrochloride (vitamin B_6), 2 mg; cyanocobalamin (vitamin B_{12}), 6 µg; folic acid, 400 µg; pantothenic acid, 10 mg; iron, 18 mg; calcium, 100 mg; phosphorus, 100 mg; magnesium, 100 mg

Comments: Accidental iron poisoning is common in children; so be sure to keep One-A-Day multivitamin plus minerals safely out of their reach.

One-A-Day multivitamin plus minerals contains ingredients which accumulate and are stored in the body. The recommended dose should not be exceeded for long periods (several weeks to months) except by physician's orders.

The iron in One-A-Day multivitamin plus minerals interacts with oral tetracycline hydrochloride and reduces the absorption of the antibiotic. Consult your pharmacist or physician.

Optilets-500 multivitamin

Manufacturer: Abbott Laboratories
Dosage Form: Tablet
Ingredients: vitamin A, 10,000 IU; vitamin D, 400 IU; vitamin E, 30 IU; sodium ascorbate (vitamin C), 500 mg; thiamine hydrochloride (vitamin B_1), 15 mg; riboflavin (vitamin B_2), 10 mg; niacinamide, 100 mg; pyridoxine hydrochloride (vitamin B_6), 5 mg; cyanocobalamin (vitamin B_{12}), 12 µg; calcium pantothenate, 20 mg

Comments: Optilets-500 multivitamin contains ingredients which accumulate and are stored in the body. The recommended dose should not be exceeded for long periods (several weeks to months) except by physician's orders.

Optilets-500 multivitamin contains vitamin B_6 which may interact with levodopa (L-Dopa).

Vitamin Supplement Profiles

Optilets-500 multivitamin may interfere with the results of urine tests. Tell your physician and pharmacist you are taking this product.

Optilets-500 multivitamin contains one or more vitamin or mineral in amounts (per tablet) greater than 100 percent of the U.S. RDA. Vitamins or minerals are not present in toxic amounts, however.

Optilets-M-500 multivitamin

Manufacturer: Abbott Laboratories
Dosage Form: Tablet
Ingredients: copper, 2 mg; zinc, 1.5 mg; manganese, 1 mg; iodine, 150 µg; vitamin A, 10,000 IU; vitamin D, 400 IU; vitamin E, 30 IU; sodium ascorbate (vitamin C), 500 mg; thiamine hydrochloride (vitamin B_1), 15 mg; riboflavin (vitamin B_2), 10 mg; niacinamide, 100 mg; pyridoxine hydrochloride (vitamin B_6), 5 mg; cyanocobalamin (vitamin B_{12}), 12 µg; calcium pantothenate, 20 mg; iron, 20 mg; magnesium, 80 mg
Comments: Accidental iron poisoning is common in children; so be sure to keep Optilets-M-500 multivitamin safely out of their reach.

Optilets-M-500 multivitamin contains ingredients which accumulate and are stored in the body. The recommended dose should not be exceeded for long periods (several weeks to months) except by physician's orders.

Optilets-M-500 contains vitamin B_6 which may interact with levodopa (L-Dopa).

The iron in Optilets-M-500 interacts with oral tetracycline hydrochloride and reduces the absorption of the antibiotic. Consult your pharmacist or physician.

Optilets-M-500 multivitamin may interfere with the results of urine tests. Tell your physician and pharmacist you are taking this product.

Optilets-M-500 multivitamin contains one or more vitamin or mineral in amounts (per tablet) greater than

Vitamin Supplement Profiles

100 percent of the U.S. RDA. Vitamins or minerals are not present in toxic amounts, however.

Paladac multivitamin

Manufacturer: Parke, Davis & Company
Dosage Form: Liquid
Ingredients: Content per 5 ml; vitamin A, 5000 IU; vitamin D, 400 IU; ascorbic acid (vitamin C), 50 mg; thiamine hydrochloride (vitamin B_1), 3 mg; riboflavin phosphate (vitamin B_2), 3 mg; niacinamide, 20 mg; pyridoxine hydrochloride (vitamin B_6), 1 mg; cyanocobalamin (vitamin B_{12}), 5 µg; sodium pantothenate, 5 mg
Comments: Paladac multivitamin contains ingredients which accumulate and are stored in the body. The recommended dose should not be exceeded for long periods (several weeks to months) except by physician's orders.

Paladac multivitamin will taste better chilled, although refrigeration is not required for its stability.

Paladac multivitamin contains one or more vitamin or mineral in amounts (per liquid measure) greater than 100 percent of the U.S. RDA. Vitamins or minerals are not toxic, however.

Paladac with Minerals multivitamin

Manufacturer: Parke, Davis & Company
Dosage Form: Chewable tablet
Ingredients: potassium sulfate, 2.5 mg; potassium iodide, 50 µg; vitamin A, 4000 IU; vitamin D, 400 IU; vitamin E, 10 IU; sodium ascorbate (vitamin C), 50 mg; thiamine mononitrate (vitamin B_1), 3 mg; riboflavin (vitamin B_2), 3 mg; niacinamide, 20 mg; pyridoxine hydrochloride (vitamin B_6), 1 mg; cyanocobalamin (vitamin B_{12}), 5 µg; calcium pantothenate, 5 mg; iron, 5 mg; calcium, 23 mg; phosphorus, 17 mg; magnesium oxide, 1 mg
Comments: Accidental iron poisoning is common in

Vitamin Supplement Profiles

children; so be sure to keep Paladac with Minerals multivitamin safely out of their reach.

Paladac with Minerals multivitamin contains ingredients which accumulate and are stored in the body. The recommended dose should not be exceeded for long periods (several weeks to months) except by physician's orders.

Chewable tablets should never be referred to as "candy" or as "candy-flavored" vitamins. Your child may take you literally and swallow toxic amounts.

The iron in Paladac with Minerals multivitamin interacts with oral tetracycline hydrochloride and reduces the absorption of the antibiotic. Consult your pharmacist or physician.

Paladac with Minerals multivitamin contains one or more vitamin or mineral in amounts (per tablet) greater than 100 percent of the U.S. RDA. Vitamins or minerals are not present in toxic amounts, however.

Poly-Vi-Sol multivitamin

Manufacturer: Mead Johnson Nutritional Division
Dosage Form: Chewable tablet
Ingredients: vitamin A, 2500 IU; vitamin D, 400 IU; vitamin E, 15 IU; ascorbic acid (vitamin C), 60 mg; thiamine (vitamin B_1), 1.05 mg; riboflavin (vitamin B_2), 1.2 mg; niacin, 13.5 mg; pyridoxine hydrochloride (vitamin B_6), 1.05 mg; cyanocobalamin (vitamin B_{12}), 4.5 μg; folic acid, 300 μg
Comments: Poly-Vi-Sol multivitamin contains ingredients which accumulate and are stored in the body. The recommended dose should not be exceeded for long periods (several weeks to months) except by physician's orders.

Chewable tablets should never be referred to as "candy" or as "candy-flavored" vitamins. Your child may take you literally and swallow toxic amounts.

Vitamin Supplement Profiles

Poly-Vi-Sol with Iron multivitamin

Manufacturer: Mead Johnson Nutritional Division
Dosage Form: Chewable tablet
Ingredients: vitamin A, 2500 IU; vitamin D, 400 IU; vitamin E, 15 IU; ascorbic acid (vitamin C), 60 mg; thiamine (vitamin B_1), 1.05 mg; riboflavin (vitamin B_2), 1.2 mg; niacin, 13.5 mg; pyridoxine hydrochloride (vitamin B_6), 1.05 mg; cyanocobalamin (vitamin B_{12}), 4.5 μg; folic acid, 300 μg; iron, 12 mg
Comments: Accidental iron poisoning is common in children, so be sure to keep Poly-Vi-Sol with Iron multivitamin safely out of their reach.

Poly-Vi-Sol with Iron multivitamin contains ingredients which accumulate and are stored in the body. The recommended dose should not be exceeded for long periods (several weeks to months) except by physician's orders.

Chewable tablets should never be referred to as "candy" or as "candy-flavored" vitamins. Your child may take you literally and swallow toxic amounts.

The iron in Poly-Vi-Sol with Iron multivitamin interacts with oral tetracycline hydrochloride and reduces the absorption of the antibiotic. Consult your pharmacist or physician.

Simron iron supplement

Manufacturer: Merrell-National Laboratories
Dosage Form: Capsule
Ingredients: ferrous gluconate, 86 mg; polysorbate 20, 400 mg
Comments: The addition of polysorbate 20 is to prevent constipation which may result from iron therapy.

Accidental iron poisoning is common in children; so be sure to keep Simron iron supplement safely out of their reach.

The iron in Simron iron supplement interacts with oral

Vitamin Supplement Profiles

tetracycline hydrochloride and reduces the absorption of the antibiotic. Consult your pharmacist or physician.

Stresscaps multivitamin

Manufacturer: Lederle Laboratories
Dosage Form: Capsule
Ingredients: ascorbic acid (vitamin C), 300 mg; thiamine (vitamin B_1), 10 mg; riboflavin (vitamin B_2), 10 mg; niacinamide, 100 mg; pyridoxine hydrochloride (vitamin B_6), 2 mg; cyanocobalamin (vitamin B_{12}), 4 µg; calcium pantothenate, 20 mg
Comments: If two or more capsules are taken daily, Stresscaps multivitamin may interfere with the results of urine tests.

Stresscaps multivitamin contains one or more vitamin or mineral in amounts (per capsule) greater than 100 percent of the U.S. RDA. Vitamins or minerals are not present in toxic amounts, however.

Stresstabs 600 multivitamin

Manufacturer: Lederle Laboratories
Dosage Form: Tablet
Ingredients: vitamin E, 30 IU; ascorbic acid (vitamin C), 600 mg; thiamine (vitamin B_1), 15 mg; riboflavin (vitamin B_2), 15 mg; niacinamide, 100 mg; pyridoxine hydrochloride (vitamin B_6), 5 mg; cyanocobalamin (vitamin B_{12}), 12 µg; calcium pantothenate, 20 mg
Comments: Stresstabs 600 multivitamin contains vitamin B_6 which may interact with levodopa (L-Dopa).

Stresstabs 600 multivitamin may interfere with the results of urine tests. Tell your physician and pharmacist you are taking this product.

Stresstabs 600 multivitamin contains one or more vitamin or mineral in amounts (per tablet) greater than 100 percent of the U.S. RDA. Vitamins or minerals are not present in toxic amounts, however.

Vitamin Supplement Profiles

Stuart Prenatal multivitamin

Manufacturer: Stuart Pharmaceuticals
Dosage Form: Tablet
Ingredients: potassium iodine, 150 µg; vitamin A, 8000 IU; vitamin D, 400 IU; vitamin E, 30 IU; ascorbic acid (vitamin C), 60 mg; thiamine (vitamin B_1), 1.7 mg; riboflavin (vitamin B_2), 2 mg; niacinamide, 20 mg; pyridoxine (vitamin B_6), 4 mg; cyanocobalamin (vitamin B_{12}), 8 µg; folic acid, 800 µg; iron, 60 mg; calcium, 200 mg; magnesium, 100 mg
Comments: This product is intended for use in pregnancy. If you think you are pregnant you should see your doctor before taking any medications.

Accidental iron poisoning is common in children; so be sure to keep Stuart Prenatal multivitamin safely out of their reach.

Stuart Prenatal multivitamin contains vitamin B_6 which may interact with levodopa (L-Dopa). This interaction occurs only if two or more doses of Stuart Prenatal multivitamin are taken each day.

The iron in Stuart Prenatal multivitamin interacts with oral tetracycline hydrochloride and reduces the absorption of the antibiotic. Consult your pharmacist or physician.

Stuart Prenatal multivitamin contains one or more vitamin or mineral in amounts (per tablet) greater than 100 percent of the U.S. RDA. Vitamins or minerals are not present in toxic amounts, however.

Super Plenamins multivitamin

Manufacturer: Rexall Drug Company
Dosage Form: Tablet
Ingredients: vitamin A, 8000 IU; vitamin D, 400 IU; vitamin E, 1.0 IU; ascorbic acid, (vitamin C), 75 mg; thiamine hydrochloride (vitamin B_1), 2.5 mg; riboflavin (vitamin B_2), 2.5 mg; niacin, 20 mg; pyridoxine hydrochloride

Vitamin Supplement Profiles

(vitamin B_6), 1 mg; cyanocobalamin (vitamin B_{12}), 3 μg; biotin, 20 μg; pantothenic acid, 3 mg; liver concentrate, 100 mg; iron, 30 mg; calcium, 75 mg; phosphorus, 58 mg; iodine, 0.15 mg; copper, 0.75 mg; manganese 1.25 mg; magnesium, 10 mg; zinc, 1 mg

Comments: Super Plenamins multivitamin contains ingredients which accumulate and are stored in the body. The recommended dose should not be exceeded for long periods (several weeks to months) except by physician's orders.

Super Plenamins multivitamin contains one or more vitamin or mineral in amounts (per tablet) greater than 100 percent of the U.S. RDA. Vitamins or minerals are not present in toxic amounts, however.

Thera-Combex H-P multivitamin

Manufacturer: Parke, Davis & Company
Dosage Form: Capsule
Ingredients: ascorbic acid (vitamin C), 500 mg; thiamine mononitrate (vitamin B_1), 25 mg; riboflavin (vitamin B_2), 15 mg; niacinamide, 100 mg; pyridoxine hydrochloride (vitamin B_6), 10 mg; cyanocobalamin (vitamin B_{12}), 5 μg; panthenol, 20 mg

Comments: Thera-Combex H-P multivitamin contains vitamin B_6 which may interact with levodopa (L-Dopa).

Thera-Combex H-P multivitamin may interfere with the results of urine tests. Tell your physician and pharmacist you are taking this product.

Thera-Combex H-P multivitamin contains one or more vitamin or mineral in amounts (per capsule) greater than 100 percent of the U.S. RDA. Vitamins or minerals are not present in toxic amounts, however.

Theragran multivitamin (liquid)

Manufacturer: E. R. Squibb & sons
Dosage Form: Liquid

Vitamin Supplement Profiles

Ingredients: Content per 5 ml: vitamin A, 10,000 IU; vitamin D, 400 IU; ascorbic acid (vitamin C), 200 mg; thiamine (vitamin B_1), 10 mg; riboflavin (vitamin B_2), 10 mg; niacinamide, 100 mg; pyridoxine hydrochloride (vitamin B_6), 5 mg; cyanocobalamin (vitamin B_{12}), 5 µg, panthenol, 20 mg

Comments: Theragran multivitamin (liquid) will taste better chilled, although refrigeration is not required for its stability.

Theragran multivitamin (liquid) contains ingredients which accumulate and are stored in the body. The recommended dose should not be exceeded for long periods (several weeks to months) except by physician's orders.

Theragran multivitamin (liquid) contains vitamin B_6 which may interact with levodopa (L-Dopa).

If two or more doses are taken daily, Theragran multivitamin (liquid) may interfere with the results of urine tests. Tell your physician and pharmacist you are taking this product.

Theragran multivitamin (liquid) contains one or more vitamin or mineral in amounts (per liquid measure) greater than 100 percent of the U.S. RDA. Vitamins or minerals are not present in toxic amounts, however.

Theragran multivitamin (tablet)

Manufacturer: E. R. Squibb & Sons
Dosage Form: Tablet
Ingredients: vitamin A, 10,000 IU; vitamin D, 400 IU; vitamin E, 15 IU; ascorbic acid (vitamin C), 200 mg; thiamine (vitamin B_1), 10 mg; riboflavin (vitamin B_2), 10 mg; niacinamide, 100 mg; pyridoxine hydrochloride (vitamin B_6), 5 mg; cyanocobalamin (vitamin B_{12}), 5 µg; calcium pantothenate, 20 mg

Comments: Theragran multivitamin (tablet) contains ingredients which accumulate and are stored in the body. The recommended dose should not be exceeded for

Vitamin Supplement Profiles

long periods (several weeks to months) except by physician's orders.

Theragran multivitamin (tablet) contains vitamin B_6 which may interact with levodopa (L-Dopa).

If two or more tablets are taken daily, Theragran multivitamin (tablet) may interfere with the results of urine tests. Tell your physician and pharmacist you are taking this product.

Theragran multivitamin (tablet) contains one or more vitamin or mineral in amounts (per tablet) greater than 100 percent of the U.S. RDA. Vitamins or minerals are not present in toxic amounts, however.

Theragran-M multivitamin

Manufacturer: E. R. Squibb & Sons
Dosage Form: Tablet
Ingredients: copper, 2 mg; zinc, 1.5 mg; manganese, 1 mg; iodine, 150 µg; vitamin A, 10,000 IU; vitamin D, 400 IU; vitamin E, 15 IU; ascorbic acid (vitamin C), 200 mg; thiamine (vitamin B_1), 10 mg; riboflavin (vitamin B_2), 10 mg; niacinamide, 100 mg; pyridoxine hydrochloride (vitamin B_6), 5 mg; cyanocobalamin (vitamin B_{12}), 5 µg; calcium pantothenate, 20 mg; iron, 12 mg; magnesium, 65 mg
Comments: Accidental iron poisoning is common in children; so be sure to keep Theragran-M multivitamin safely out of their reach.

Theragran-M multivitamin contains ingredients which accumulate and are stored in the body. The recommended dose should not be exceeded for long periods (several weeks to months) except by physician's orders.

Theragran-M multivitamin contains vitamin B_6 which may interact with levodopa (L-Dopa).

The iron in Theragran-M multivitamin interacts with oral tetracycline hydrochloride and reduces the absorption of the antibiotic. Consult your pharmacist or physician.

Vitamin Supplement Profiles

If two or more tablets are taken daily, Theragran-M multivitamin may interfere with the results of urine tests. Tell your physician and pharmacist you are taking this product.

Theragran-M multivitamin contains one or more vitamin or mineral in amounts (per tablet) greater than 100 percent of the U.S. RDA. Vitamins or minerals are not present in toxic amounts, however.

Tri-Vi-Sol multivitamin

Manufacturer: Mead Johnson Nutritional Division
Dosage Forms: Drop; chewable tablet
Ingredients: Content per 0.6 ml (drop); vitamin A, 900 IU; vitamin D, 240 IU; ascorbic acid (vitamin C), 21 mg. Chewable tablet: vitamin A, 2500 IU; vitamin D, 400 IU; ascorbic acid (vitamin C), 60 mg
Comments: Tri-Vi-Sol multivitamin drops will taste better chilled, although refrigeration is not required for its stability.

Tri-Vi-Sol multivitamin contains ingredients which accumulate and are stored in the body. The recommended dose should not be exceeded for long periods (several weeks to months) except by physician's orders.

Chewable tablets should never be referred to as "candy" or as "candy-flavored" vitamins. Your child may take you literally and swallow toxic amounts.

Tri-Vi-sol with Iron multivitamin

Manufacturer: Mead Johnson Nutritional Division
Dosage Form: Drop
Ingredients: Content per 1 ml: vitamin A, 1500 IU; vitamin D, 400 IU; ascorbic acid (vitamin C), 35 mg; iron, 10 mg
Comments: Accidental iron poisoning is common in children; so be sure to keep Tri-Vi-Sol with Iron multivitamin safely out of their reach.

Tri-Vi-Sol with Iron multivitamin will taste better chilled,

Vitamin Supplement Profiles

although refrigeration is not required for its stability.

Tri-Vi-Sol with Iron multivitamin contains ingredients which accumulate and are stored in the body. The recommended dose should not be exceeded for long periods (several weeks to months) except by physician's orders.

The iron in Tri-Vi-Sol with Iron multivitamin interacts with oral tetracycline hydrochloride and reduces the absorption of the antibiotic. Consult your pharmacist or physician.

Unicap multivitamin (capsule)

Manufacturer: The Upjohn Company
Dosage Form: Capsule
Ingredients: vitamin A, 5000 IU; vitamin D, 400 IU; vitamin E, 15 IU; ascorbic acid (vitamin C), 60 mg; thiamine hydrochloride (vitamin B_1), 1.5 mg; riboflavin (vitamin B_2), 1.7 mg; niacinamide, 20 mg; pyridoxine hydrochloride (vitamin B_6), 2 mg; cyanocobalamin, (vitamin B_{12}), 6 µg; folic acid, 0.4 mg
Comments: Unicap multivitamin (capsule) contains ingredients which accumulate and are stored in the body. The recommended dose should not be exceeded for long periods (several weeks to months) except by physician's orders.

Unicap multivitamin (chewable tablet; tablet)

Manufacturer: The Upjohn Company
Dosage Forms: Chewable tablet; tablet
Ingredients: vitamin A, 5000 IU; vitamin D, 400 IU; ascorbic acid (vitamin C), 60 mg; thiamine mononitrate (vitamin B_1), 1.5 mg; riboflavin (vitamin B_2), 1.7 mg; niacin, 20 mg; pyridoxine hydrochloride (vitamin B_6), 2 mg; cyanocobalamin (vitamin B_{12}), 6 µg; folic acid, 0.4 mg
Comments: Unicap multivitamin (chewable tablet and

Vitamin Supplement Profiles

tablet) contains ingredients which accumulate and are stored in the body. The recommended dose should not be exceeded for long periods (several weeks to months) except by physician's orders.

Chewable tablets should never be referred to as "candy" or as "candy-flavored" vitamins.

Unicap M multivitamin

Manufacturer: The Upjohn Company
Dosage Form: Tablet
Ingredients: vitamin A, 5000 IU; vitamin D, 400 IU; vitamin E, 10 IU; thiamine (vitamin B_1), 2.5 mg; riboflavin (vitamin B_2), 2.5 mg; niacinamide, 20 mg; pantothenate, 5 mg; pyridoxine hydrochloride (vitamin B_6), 0.5 mg; cyanocobalamin (vitamin B_{12}), 2 µg; ascorbic acid (vitamin C), 50 mg; iron, 10 mg; calcium, 35 mg. Unicap M multivitamin also contains trace quantities of iodine, copper, manganese, magnesium, and potassium.
Comments: Accidental iron poisoning is common in children; so be sure to keep Unicap M multivitamin safely out of their reach.

Unicap M multivitamin contains ingredients which accumulate and are stored in the body. The recommended dose should not be exceeded for long periods (several weeks to months) except by physician's orders.

The iron in Unicap M multivitamin interacts with oral tetracycline hydrochloride and reduces the absorption of the antibiotic. Consult your pharmacist or physician.

Unicap M multivitamin contains one or more vitamin or mineral in amounts (per tablet) greater than 100 percent of the U.S. RDA. Vitamins or minerals are not present in toxic amounts, however.

Unicap Therapeutic multivitamin

Manufacturer: The Upjohn Company
Dosage Form: Tablet

Vitamin Supplement Profiles

Ingredients: potassium sulfate, 5 mg; copper sulfate, 1 mg; manganese sulfate, 1 mg; potassium iodide, 150 µg; vitamin A, 5000 IU; vitamin D, 400 IU; vitamin E, 15 IU; ascorbic acid (vitamin C), 300 mg; thiamine mononitrate (vitamin B_1), 10 mg; riboflavin (vitamin B_2), 10 mg; niacin, 100 mg; pyridoxine hydrochloride (vitamin B_6), 6 mg; cyanocobalamin (vitamin B_{12}), 18 µg; pantothenic acid, 10 mg; iron, 18 mg; zinc, 15 mg; potassium, 5 mg

Comments: Accidental iron poisoning is common in children; so be sure to keep Unicap Therapeutic multivitamin safely out of their reach.

Unicap Therapeutic multivitamin contains ingredients which accumulate and are stored in the body. The recommended dose should not be exceeded for long periods (several weeks to months) except by physician's orders.

The iron in Unicap Therapeutic multivitamin interacts with oral tetracycline hydrochloride and reduces the absorption of the antibiotic. Consult your pharmacist or physician.

If two or more tablets are taken daily, Unicap Therapeutic multivitamin may interfere with the results of urine tests. Tell your physician and pharmacist you are taking this product.

Unicap Therapeutic multivitamin contains one or more vitamin or mineral in amounts (per tablet) greater than 100 percent of the U.S. RDA. Vitamins or minerals are not present in toxic amounts, however.

Vi-Penta Infant Drops multivitamin

Manufacturer: Roche Products Inc.
Dosage Form: Drop
Ingredients: Content per 0.6 ml: vitamin A, 5000 IU; vitamin D, 400 IU; vitamin E, 2 IU; ascorbic acid (vitamin C), 50 mg
Comments: Vi-Penta Infant Drops multivitamin contains ingredients which accumulate and are stored in the

Vitamin Supplement Profiles

body. The recommended dose should not be exceeded for long periods (several weeks to months) except by physician's orders.

Vi-Penta Infant Drops multivitamin will taste better chilled, although refrigeration is not required for its stability.

Vi-Penta Infant Drops multivitamin contains one or more vitamin or mineral in amounts (per liquid measure) greater than 100 percent of the U.S. RDA for infants and children less than 4 years of age. Vitamins or minerals are not present in toxic amounts, however.

Vi-Penta multivitamin

Manufacturer: Roche Products, Inc.
Dosage Form: Drop
Ingredients: Content per 0.6 ml: biotin, 30 μg; vitamin A, 5000 IU; vitamin D, 400 IU; vitamin E, 2 IU; ascorbic acid (vitamin C), 50 mg; thiamine hydrochloride (vitamin B_1), 1 mg; riboflavin (vitamin B_2), 1 mg; niacinamide, 10 mg; pyridoxine hydrochloride (vitamin B_6), 1 mg; panthenol, 10 mg
Comments: Vi-Penta multivitamin contains ingredients which accumulate and are stored in the body. The recommended dose should not be exceeded for long periods (several weeks to months) except by physician's orders.

Vi-Penta multivitamin will taste better chilled, although refrigeration is not required for its stability.

Zymalixir multivitamin

Manufacturer: The Upjohn Company
Dosage Form: Syrup
Ingredients: Content per 5 ml: liver concentrate, 65 mg; alcohol, 1.5%; thiamine hydrochloride (vitamin B_1), 1 mg; riboflavin (vitamin B_2), 1 mg; niacinamide, 8 mg; pyridoxine hydrochloride (vitamin B_6), 0.5 mg; cyanoco-

Vitamin Supplement Profiles

balamin (vitamin B_{12}), 2 μg; iron, 15 mg
Comments: Accidental iron poisoning is common in children; so be sure to keep Zymalixir multivitamin safely out of their reach.

Because Zymalixir multivitamin contains alcohol, do not take this product if you are taking Antabuse antialcohol preparation.

Zymalixir multivitamin will taste better chilled, although refrigeration is not required for its stability.

The iron in Zymalixir multivitamin interacts with oral tetracycline hydrochloride and reduces the absorption of the antibiotic. Consult your pharmacist or doctor.

Zymasyrup multivitamin

Manufacturer: The Upjohn Company
Dosage Form: Syrup
Ingredients: Content per 5 ml: alcohol, 2%, vitamin A, 5000 IU; vitamin D, 400 IU; ascorbic acid (vitamin C), 60 mg; thiamine hydrochloride (vitamin B_1), 1 mg; riboflavin (vitamin B_2), 1 mg; niacinamide, 10 mg; pyridoxine hydrochloride (vitamin B_6), 0.5 mg; cyanocobalamin (vitamin B_{12}), 3 μg; panthenol, 3.0 mg
Comments: Zymasyrup multivitamin contains ingredients which accumulate and are stored in the body. The recommended dose should not be exceeded for long periods (several weeks to months) except by physician's orders.

Because Zymasyrup multivitamin contains alcohol, do not take this product if you are taking Antabuse antialcohol preparation.

Zymasyrup multivitamin will taste better chilled, although refrigeration is not required for its stability.

Glossary

absorption: Passage of nutrients and other food components through the walls of the small intestine into the body.
amino acids: Organic compounds from which proteins are made.
anemia: Condition in which there is a lower than normal amount of hemoglobin and/or red blood cells.
antagonist: Compound which interferes with the normal action of a vitamin.
antioxidant: Substance which protects other substances from being oxidized.
antirachitic: Property of providing protection against development of rickets. Vitamin D is the antirachitic vitamin.
antiscorbutic: Property of protecting against the development of scurvy. Ascorbic acid (vitamin C) is the antiscorbutic vitamin.
antivitamin: Compound which destroys or interferes with the normal action of a vitamin.
apoenzyme: The protein portion of an enzyme.
arteriosclerosis: Condition in which the walls of the arteries are thickened and hardened.
ascorbic acid: Vitamin C.

Glossary

atherosclerosis: Type of arteriosclerosis in which there are deposits of fats and cholesterol on blood vessel walls.
avidin: Substance in raw egg white which combines with biotin making the vitamin unavailable for absorption.
Basic Four: Food selection plan based on four classes of foods: meats, milk, fruits and vegetables, and cereal products.
beriberi: Disease caused by thiamin deficiency.
bile: Secretion made by the liver, stored in the gall bladder, and delivered to the small intestine where it is necessary for digestion and absorption of fats and fat-soluble vitamins.
biotin: One of the B vitamins.
blood plasma: Colorless water solution remaining when red blood cells are removed from the blood.
blood serum: Colorless water solution remaining when red blood cells and the clotting proteins are removed from the blood.
calorie: Unit of heat energy used to express the energy value of food.
carbohydrates: One of the major classes of essential nutrients. Starches and sugars are the carbohydrates in foods. Used primarily as source of energy.
carotenes: Orange-yellow pigments, many of which can be changed in the body to vitamin A. Provitamin A compounds.
catalyst: Substances which change the speed of a chemical reaction. Enzymes are organic catalysts.
cheilosis: Condition characterized by cracks at corners of the mouth and sore lips. Sometimes seen in riboflavin deficiency.
cholecalciferol: Vitamin D_3.
cholesterol: One of a class of lipids called sterols. Present only in animal tissues. Provided by diets containing animal foods and also synthesized in the body. Essential component of cell membranes.
coenzyme: Organic compound (often a vitamin) which combines with a protein (apoenzyme) to form an active enzyme.
collagen: Sometimes called "cell cement." One of the proteins making up connective tissues.
compound: Substance composed of two or more elements.
connective tissue: Body tissue which holds cells and other tissues together to give form and structure to body organs.
cyanocobalamin: Vitamin B_{12}.
deficiency: Condition produced when an essential nutrient is not supplied to the body in amounts adequate to meet requirements.
delirium: Mental condition characterized by restlessness, excitability, confusion, and delusions.
dermatitis: Inflammation, soreness of the skin.
diet:
    purified: Composed of isolated preparations of the essential nutrients rather than of ordinary foods.

Glossary

mixed: Composed of a variety of foods of different classes (e.g., meats, milk products, cereals, fruits and vegetables).
digestion: Process by which foods are broken down and prepared for absorption.
DNA (deoxyribonucleic acid): Material in cells containing the genes.
element: Substance composed of only one kind of atom. Elements are the basic units making up all matter, animate and inanimate.
enzymes: Organic catalysts which speed up chemical reactions in plants and animals.
enrichment: Addition of nutrients to foods, e.g., thiamin, riboflavin, niacin and iron to cereal products.
epithelium: Type of body tissue including the skin and the linings of the respiratory tract and the digestive system.
essential amino acids: Those amino acids of proteins which cannot be made in the body; must be supplied by the diet.
essential nutrients: Substances which are necessary for the normal function of body processes for good health. They cannot be made in the body and must come from foods.
fats: One of the major classes of essential nutrients. Not soluble in water. Used principally as a source of energy. Also called lipids.
fatty acids: Organic compounds which are the major components of fats and oils.
fetus: Unborn young of animals during late stages of development.
folacin: One of the B vitamins.
Food and Drug Administration (FDA): Government agency responsible for regulation of foods and drugs, to ensure their safety for the protection of the consumer. The agency enforces the Federal Food, Drug and Cosmetic Act.
Food and Nutrition Board (of the National Academy of Sciences—National Research Council): Group of nutrition experts working to encourage good food use practices. The Board established the Recommended Dietary Allowances (RDAs) for essential nutrients, adding to and revising the list of allowances as scientific information becomes available.
fortification: Addition of a nutrient to a food which normally contains little or none of the nutrient, e.g., addition of vitamin D to milk.
Four Food Groups: Basis of the U.S.D.A.'s Daily Food Guide, which suggests inclusion in each day's diet of foods from four different food classes—meats, milk and dairy products, fruits and vegetables, and cereal foods.
fructose: A sugar or simple carbohydrate present in small amounts in some foods. Makes up half of sucrose (table sugar).
glucose: Sugar or simple carbohydrate. The sugar of the blood. Makes up half of sucrose (table sugar).
glycogen: Storage form of carbohydrate in body.

Glossary

hemoglobin: Red pigment in red blood cells. Carries oxygen from lungs to other parts of the body.
hemorrhage: Loss of blood.
hormones: Organic compounds made by special glands. Regulate many body processes.
hypervitaminosis: Excessive storage of vitamins in the body, especially of vitamins A and D.
ileum: Lower part of the small intestine.
intake: Consumption of foods and nutrients.
international unit (IU): Used instead of metric values (e.g., milligrams or micrograms) to express requirements for and food contents of vitamins A, D, and E.
intrinsic factor: Compound produced in the stomach of normal people. It is necessary for the absorption of vitamin B_{12}. People with pernicious anemia cannot make intrinsic factor.
isolate: Refers to separation from a complex mixture of a substance in pure form (e.g., isolation of a vitamin from a food).
lipids: See **fats**.
macrocytic anemia: Type of anemia in which red blood cells are larger than normal. Seen in folacin and vitamin B_{12} deficiencies.
macroelement: Mineral needed by humans in amounts greater than 100 mg per day.
malabsorption: Condition in which absorption of nutrients from the intestinal tract is impaired and reduced.
megadose: Large daily dose or intake of a vitamin, usually at least ten times higher than the recommended allowance.
megaloblastic anemia: Type of anemia characterized by abnormally large and immature red blood cells. Seen in folacin and vitamin B_{12} deficiencies.
megavitamin therapy: Use of large doses of vitamins for the prevention, treatment, or cure of physical or mental disorders.
metabolism: All of the chemical reactions involved in the functioning of the body.
microcytic anemia: Type of anemia in which red blood cells are smaller than normal. Seen in iron deficiency.
microelement: Mineral needed by humans in amounts less than 100 mg per day.
microorganisms: Tiny, one-cell living things such as bacteria and yeast.
mucosa: Membrane of epithelial tissue lining the digestive and respiratory tracts.
multivitamin: Description of supplements containing two or more vitamins.
nausea: Sick at the stomach; usually with vomiting.
niacin: One of the B vitamins. Sometimes called vitamin B_3.

Glossary

niacinamide: One form of niacin. The compound included in vitamin supplements.
nicotinic acid: One form of niacin.
night blindness: Reduced ability to adapt to changes in light and to see in dim light.
nutrient: Component of foods which, after digestion and absorption, is used for energy, growth, and maintenance of the body or for regulation of body processes.
nutrition: The science of foods—their composition, digestion, absorption, and use in the metabolism of the body.
nyctalopia: Night blindness.
orthomolecular therapy: Use of large amounts of vitamins, usually for the prevention or treatment of mental disorders.
osteomalacia: Vitamin D deficiency in adults characterized by loss of calcium from the bones.
OTC (over-the-counter): Products marketed as drugs but available without a physician's prescription.
overage: Practice of adding more than the labeled amount of a vitamin to a fortified food or a supplement to allow for gradual loss of the vitamin thus ensuring that the product will provide the labeled amount of the vitamin throughout its expected shelf-life.
overdose: Intake of a vitamin in an amount large enough to be toxic or to cause adverse side effects.
oxidation: Combination with oxygen (or loss of hydrogen) to change the chemical structure of a compound.
pantothenic acid: One of the B vitamins.
pellagra: Disease produced by severe deficiency of niacin.
pernicious anemia: An inherited disease characterized by the inability to make intrinsic factor.
plasma: The liquid portion of blood (see **blood plasma**).
polyneuritis: Inflammation of the nerves, as in severe thiamin deficiency.
polyunsaturated fatty acids: Fatty acids which have less than the maximum amount of hydrogen in their molecular structure, making them susceptible to oxidation.
protein: One of the major classes of essential nutrients. Made up of amino acids. Used primarily for building and maintaining body tissues, but can furnish energy.
provitamin: A compound which does not have vitamin activity, but which can be changed in the body into an active form of a vitamin.
pyridoxine: Vitamin B_6.
RDA (Recommended Dietary Allowance): Food and Nutrition Board's suggested daily intake of an essential nutrient. Nutrient intakes in amounts approximating the RDAs will meet the requirements of essentially all normal, healthy individuals.

Glossary

rancid: Having unpleasant odor and taste, as fats and oils which have been oxidized.
retinal: Form of vitamin A present in the retina of the eye which functions to permit seeing in dim light.
retinol: Vitamin A.
riboflavin: Vitamin B_2.
rickets: Disease produced by severe deficiency of vitamin D. Characterized by poor development of bones.
scurvy: Disease produced by severe deficiency of vitamin C.
serum: Clear liquid which separates from clotted blood (See **blood serum**).
subclinical deficiency: Condition produced by a low intake of a vitamin. It can be detected only by laboratory tests, since outward, visible signs or symptoms of deficiency are not present.
supplement: In nutrition, the addition of a nutrient or nutrients to ordinary diets.
symptom: An abnormal condition which indicates the presence of a disorder or disease (e.g., vitamin-deficiency symptom).
syndrome: Group of symptoms which occur together.
synthesis: Process by which a substance is manufactured or made in the body; often a complex substance made from simple starting materials.
therapeutic: Applies to the use of vitamin supplements as drugs for the prevention or correction of a deficiency of the vitamin, or for the management of a disease or disorder unrelated to a deficiency.
thiamin: Vitamin B_1.
tocopherol: A compound with vitamin E activity.
toxicity: The quality or condition of being harmful or poisonous.
tryptophan: One of the amino acids, which are the compounds making up proteins. In addition to its many other functions, tryptophan is a provitamin, since the body can change it to niacin.
ultraviolet rays: Light rays with wavelengths shorter than those of visible light.
U.S. RDA (United States Recommended Daily Allowances): Standards established by the Food and Drug Administration for use in providing nutrition information on food labels. The values were based on the Food and Nutrition Board's RDAs (Recommended Dietary Allowances), but they are not the same.
vascular: Refers to blood vessels.
visual purple: Pigment in retina of the eye, containing retinal, which allows seeing in dim light.
vitamin: Organic compound, which is rarely synthesized in the body. Needed in small amounts and must be supplied by the diet.
vitamin activity: Refers to the value of a food as a source of a specific vitamin, especially when the food contains several different forms of

Glossary

a vitamin or contains a provitamin.

vitamin B$_3$: Niacin. Designation seldom used today by nutritionists.

vitamin B$_5$: Pantothenic acid. Designation seldom used today.

vitamin B$_{15}$: Pangamic acid. Not recognized as a vitamin for humans.

vitamin B$_{17}$: Laetrile. Controversial anticancer substance definitely not recognized as a vitamin.

vitamin content: The amount of a vitamin in a diet or in a specified quantity of food.

vitamin derivative: Compounds produced in the body from vitamins. Some derivatives are the biologically active forms of the vitamin.

vitamin F: Unsaturated fatty acids. Some of these are essential nutrients, but they are not classified by nutritionists as vitamins.

vitamin P: Bioflavonoids, including rutin and hesperidin. Not recognized as vitamins for humans.

vitamin potency: Refers usually to the amount of a vitamin in a commercially available supplement.

vitamin Q: Compound claimed to aid in blood clotting. Not recognized as a vitamin for humans.

vitamin U: Metenoic acid, supposedly beneficial in treatment of ulcers. Not recognized as a vitamin for humans.

xerophthalmia: Eye damage caused by vitamin A deficiency; may lead to blindness.

Bibliography

Callahan, D., and Payne, A.S. *The Great Nutrition Puzzle.* New York: Charles Scribner's Sons, 1956.

Chaney, M.S., Ross, M.L., and Witschi, J.D. *Nutrition,* 9th ed. Boston: Houghton Mifflin Company, 1979.

Davidson, S., et al. *Human Nutrition and Dietetics,* 6th ed. London: Churchill Livingston, 1975.

Dykes, M.H.M., and Meier, P. "Ascorbic Acid and the Common Cold. Evaluation of its Efficacy and Toxicity." *Journal of the American Medical Association,* Vol. 231 (1975), pp. 1073-1079.

The Fat-Soluble Vitamins, ed. H.F. DeLuca, and J.W. Suttie. Madison: The University of Wisconsin Press, 1970.

Food and Drug Administration. "Vitamin and Mineral Drug Products for Over-the-Counter Human Use," *Federal Register,* Vol. 44 (March 16, 1979), pp. 16126-16201.

Herbert, V. "Megavitamin Therapy: Facts and Fiction." *Food & Nutrition News,* Vol. 47, No. 4 (March-April). Chicago: National Live Stock and Meat Board, 1976.

McCollum, E.V., *A History of Nutrition.* Boston: Houghton Mifflin Company, 1957.

Megavitamin and Orthomolecular Therapy in Psychiatry. Report of The American Psychiatric Association Task Force on Vitamin Therapy in Psychiatry. Washington, D.C.: American Psychiatric Association, 1973.

Bibliography

Modern Nutrition in Health and Disease, 5th ed., ed. R.S. Goodhart, and M.S. Shils. Philadelphia: Lea & Febiger, 1973.

Nutrition Review's Present Knowledge in Nutrition, 4th ed. New York: The Nutrition Foundation, Inc., 1976.

Preliminary Findings of the First Health and Nutrition Examination Survey, United States, 1971-72. Dietary Intake and Biochemical Findings; Anthropometric and Clinical Findings. Health Resources Administration, U.S. Dept. Health, Education and Welfare, National Center for Health Statistics, DHEW (HRA) 74-1919-1 (1974); (HRA) 75-1229 (1975).

Recommended Dietary Allowances, 8th ed. Food and Nutrition Board, National Research Council. Washington, D.C.: National Academy of Sciences, 1974.

Roe, D.A. *Drug-Induced Nutritional Deficiencies.* Westport, CT: The AVI Publishing Company, Inc., 1976.

Second Conference on Vitamin C, ed. C.G. King, and J.J. Burns. Annals of the New York Academy of Sciences, Vol. 258, 1975.

The Ten-State Nutrition Survey, 1968-1970. DHEW (HSM) 72-8130, 72-8131, 72-8133, and 72-8134 (1972).

"The Use and Abuse of Vitamin A." Joint Committee Statement of American Academy of Pediatrics Committee on Drugs and on Nutrition. *Pediatrics,* Vol. 48 (1971), p. 655.

"Vitamin C and the Common Cold." Statement of American Academy of Pediatrics Committee on Drugs. *Newsletter of the American Academy of Pediatrics* 22 (Nov. 1, 1971).

"Vitamin E," A Scientific Status Summary by the Institute of Food Technologists' Expert Panel on Food Safety & Nutrition and The Committee on Public Information. *Nutrition Review,* Vol. 35 (1977), p. 57.

"Vitamin E—Miracle or Myth?" *FDA Consumer,* U.S. Dept. Health, Education and Welfare (July-August 1973).

"Vitamin-Mineral Safety, Toxicity, and Misuse." Report of the Committee on Safety, Toxicity, and Misuse of Vitamins and Trace Minerals. Chicago: National Nutrition Consortium, Inc. American Dietetic Association, 1978.

"Zen Macrobiotic Diets." Statement of the American Medical Association Council on Foods and Nutrition. *Journal of the American Medical Association,* Vol. 218 (1971), p. 397.

Suggested Reading

Barrett, S., and Knight, G. *The Health Robbers.* Philadelphia: George F. Stickley Company, 1976.

Deutsch, Ronald M. *The Family Guide to Better Food and Better Health.* Des Moines: Meredith Corp., 1971.

Deutsch, Ronald M. *Realities of Nutrition.* Palo Alto, CA: Bull Publishing Company, 1977.

Deutsch, Ronald M. *The New Nuts Among the Berries.* Palo Alto, CA: Bull Publishing Company, 1977.

Lowenberg, M., et al. *Food and Man,* 2nd ed. New York: John Wiley & Sons, 1974.

Nutrition Labeling, How it Can Work for You. The National Nutrition Consortium, Inc. Bethesda, MD: 1975.

Nutrition References and Book Reviews, revised 1975. The Chicago Nutrition Association. Chicago: 1975.

Stare, F.J. and McWilliams, M. *Living Nutrition,* 2nd ed. New York: John Wiley & Sons, 1977.

Stare, F.J. and Whelan, E.M. *Eat OK—Feel OK.* N. Quincy, MA: The Christopher Publishing House, 1978.

Whelan, E.M. and Stare, F.J. *Panic in the Pantry: Food Facts, Fads and Fallacies.* New York: Atheneum, 1977.

White, P.L. and Selvey, N. *Let's Talk About Food.* Acton, MA: Publishing Sciences Group, Inc., 1974.

References

The Story of Vitamins

1. Adelle Davis, *Let's Eat Right To Keep Fit* (New York: Harcourt Brace Jovanovich, Inc., 1970).
2. Linda Clark, *Linda Clark's Handbook of Natural Remedies for Common Ailments* (New York: Pocket Books, 1977).

Thiamin (Vitamin B$_1$)

1. Robert R. Williams, *Toward the Conquest of Beriberi* (Cambridge: Harvard University Press, 1961).
2. Food and Nutrition Board, National Research Council, *Recommended Dietary Allowances* (Washington, D.C.: National Academy of Sciences, 1974).
3. Food and Drug Administration, "Vitamin and Mineral Drug Products for Over-the-Counter Human Use," *Federal Register,* Vol. 44 (March 16, 1979), pp. 16126-16201.

Riboflavin (Vitamin B$_2$)

1. W.H. Sebrell and R.E. Butler, "Riboflavin Deficiency in Man: Preliminary Note," *U.S. Public Health Report,* Vol. 53 (1938), p. 2282.
2. M.K. Horwitt et al., "Effects of Dietary Depletion of Riboflavin," *Journal of Nutrition,* Vol. 39 (1949), p. 357.
3. Adelle Davis, *Let's Eat Right to Keep Fit* (New York: Harcourt Brace Jovanovich, Inc., 1970).

Niacin

1. Food and Drug Administration, "Vitamin and Mineral Drug Products for Over-the-Counter Human Use," *Federal Register,* Vol. 44 (March 16, 1979), pp. 16126-16201 (Niacin: pp. 16150-16152).
2. The Coronary Drug Project Research Group, "Clofibrate and Niacin in Coronary Heart Disease," *Journal of the American Medical Association,* Vol. 321 (1975), p. 360.

References

3. American Psychiatric Association Task Force on Vitamin Therapy in Psychiatry, *Megavitamin and Orthomolecular Therapy in Psychiatry* (Washington, D.C.: Publications Services Division, American Psychiatric Association, 1973).
4. Richard A. Passwater, *Supernutrition—Megavitamin Revolution* (New York: Pocket Books, 1976).
5. E. Cheraskin, W.M. Ringsdorf, Jr., and A. Brecher, *Psychodietetics: Food As the Key to Emotional Health* (New York: Stein and Day, 1974).

Pantothenic Acid

1. Adelle Davis, *Let's Eat Right to Keep Fit* (New York: Harcourt Brace Jovanovich, Inc., 1970).
2. Richard A. Passwater, *Supernutrition—Megavitamin Revolution* (New York: Pocket Books, 1976).
3. Linda Clark, *Linda Clark's Handbook of Natural Remedies for Common Ailments* (New York: Pocket Books, 1977).
4. Roger J. Williams, *Nutrition Against Disease* (New York: Bantam Books, 1973).

Vitamin B_6 (Pyridoxine)

1. Food and Nutrition Board, National Research Council, *Proposed Fortification Policy for Cereal-Grain Products* (Washington, D.C.: National Academy of Sciences, 1974).
2. J. E. Canham et al., "Dietary Protein—Its Relationship to Vitamin B_6 Requirements and Function," (Annapolis: New York Academy of Science, Vol. 166, 1969, p. 16).
3. L.T. Miller and H.M. Linkswiler, "Effect of Protein Intake on the Development of Abnormal Tryptophan Metabolism by Men During Vitamin B_6 Depletion," *Journal of Nutrition,* Vol. 93 (1967), p. 53.
4. Committee on Nutrition of the Mother and Preschool Child, Food and Nutrition Board, National Research Council-National Academy of Sciences, "Statement—Oral Contraceptives and Nutrition," *Journal of the American Dietetic Association,* Vol. 68 (1976), p. 419.
5. D.B. Coursin, "Convulsive Seizures in Infants with Pyridoxine-Deficient Diet," *Journal of the American Medical Association*, Vol. 154 (1954), p. 406.
6. C.J. Molony and A.H. Parmelee, "Convulsions in Young Infants as a Result of Pyridoxine (Vitamin B_6) Deficiency," *Journal of the American Medical Association*, Vol. 154 (1954), p. 405.
7. W.W. Hawkins and J. Barsky, "An Experiment on Human Vitamin B_6 Deprivation," *Science*, Vol. 108 (1948), p. 284.
8. J.F. Mueller and R.W. Vilter, "Pyridoxine Deficiency in Human

References

Beings Induced with Deoxypyridoxine," *Journal of Clinical Investigation*, Vol. 29 (1950), p. 193.
9. H. Linkswiler, "Biochemical and Physiological Changes in Vitamin B$_6$ Deficiency," *American Journal of Clinical Nutrition*, Vol. 20 (1967), p. 547.
10. Food and Drug Administration, "Vitamin and Mineral Drug Products for Over-the-Counter Human Use," *Federal Register*, Vol. 44 (March 16, 1979), pp. 16126-16201 (Vitamin B$_6$: pp. 16155-16159).
11. Daphne A. Roe, *Drug-Induced Nutritional Deficiencies* (Westport, CT: The AVI Publishing Company, Inc., 1976).
12. Adelle Davis, *Let's Eat Right to Keep Fit* (New York: Harcourt Brace Jovanovich, Inc., 1970).

Biotin

1. Food and Drug Administration, "Vitamin and Mineral Drug Products for Over-the-Counter Human Use," *Federal Register,* Vol. 44 (March 16, 1979), pp. 16126-16201 (Biotin: pp. 16143-16144).
2. Richard A. Passwater, *Supernutrition—Megavitamin Revolution* (New York: Pocket Books, 1976).
3. Catharyn Elwood, *Feel Like a Million* (New York: Pocket Books, 1965).

Folacin

1. Food and Drug Administration, "Vitamin and Mineral Drug Products for Over-the-Counter Human Use," *Federal Register*, Vol. 44 (March 16, 1979), pp. 16126-16201 (Folacin: pp. 16148-16150).
2. Richard A. Passwater, *Supernutrition—Megavitamin Revolution* (New York: Pocket Books, 1976).
3. E. Cheraskin, W.M. Ringsdorf Jr., and A. Brecher, *Psychodietetics· Food As the Key to Emotional Health* (New York: Stein and Day 1974).
4. Committee on Nutrition of the Mother and Preschool Child, Food and Nutrition Board, National Research Council-National Academy of Sciences, "Statement—Oral Contraceptives and Nutrition,"*Journal of the American Dietetic Association,* Vol. 68 (1976), p. 419.
5. Roger J. Williams, *Nutrition Against Disease* (New York: Bantam Books, 1973).

Vitamin B$_{12}$ (Cyanocobalamin)

1. Adelle Davis, *Let's Eat Right to Keep Fit* (New York: Harcourt Brace Jovanovich, Inc., 1970).
2. V. Herbert, "Vitamin B$_{12}$," *Nutrition Reviews' Present Knowledge in*

References

Nutrition, 4th ed. (Washington, D.C.: The Nutrition Foundation, 1976).

Vitamin C (Ascorbic Acid)

1. L. Pauling, *Vitamin C and the Common Cold* (San Francisco: W.H. Freeman and Co., 1970).
2. *Lind's Treatise on Scurvy*, ed. C.P. Stewart and D. Guthrie (Edinburgh: Edinburgh University Press, 1953).
3. C.G. King and W.A. Waugh, *Science*, Vol. 75 (1932), p. 357.
4. J.L. Svirbely and A. Szent-Gyorgyi, *Biochemistry Journal*, Vol. 26 (1932), p. 865.
5. National Nutrition Consortium, Inc., "Vitamin-Mineral Safety, Toxicity, and Misuse," *Report of the Committee on Safety, Toxicity, and Misuse of Vitamins and Trace Minerals*. (Chicago: The American Dietetic Association, 1978).
6. V. Herbert, "Megavitamin Therapy: Facts and Fictions," *Food and Nutrition News*, Vol. 47 (Chicago: National Live Stock and Meat Board, March-April 1976).
7. Richard A. Passwater, *Supernutrition—Megavitamin Revolution* (New York: Dial Press, 1975).
8. E. Cheraskin, W.M. Ringsdorf Jr., and A. Brecher, *Psychodietetics: Food As the Key to Emotional Health* (New York: Stein and Day, 1974).
9. Food and Drug Administration, "Vitamin and Mineral Drug Products for Over-the-Counter Human Use," *Federal Register*, Vol. 44 (March 16, 1979), pp. 16126-16201 (Vitamin C: pp. 16140-16143).
10. J.Z. Miller et al., "Therapeutic Effect of Vitamin C—A Co-twin Control Study," *Journal of the American Medical Association,* Vol. 237 (1977), p. 248.
11. T.W. Anderson, D.B.W. Reid, and G.H. Beaton, "Vitamin C and the Common Cold: A Double-blind Trial," *Canadian Medical Association Journal*, Vol. 107 (1972), p. 503.
12. T.W. Anderson, G. Suranyi, and G.H. Beaton, "The Effect on Winter Illness of Large Doses of Vitamin C," *Canadian Medical Association Journal*, Vol. 111 (1974), pp. 31-36.
13. J.L. Coulehan et al., "Vitamin C Prophylaxis in a Boarding School," *New England Journal of Medicine*, Vol. 290 (1974), p. 6.
14. J.L. Coulehan et al., "Vitamin C and Upper Respiratory Illness in Navaho Children: Preliminary Observations," *Second Conference on Vitamin C* ed. C.G. King and J.J. Burns (New York: New York Academy of Sciences, 1975).
15. J.L. Coulehan et al., "Vitamin C and Acute Illness in Navaho School Children," *New England Journal of Medicine*, Vol. 295 (1976), p. 973.

References

16. T.R. Karlowski et al., "Ascorbic Acid for the Common Cold," *Journal of the American Medical Association,* Vol. 231 (1975), p. 1038.
17. M.H.M. Dykes and P. Meier, "Ascorbic Acid and the Common Cold. Evaluation of its Efficacy and Toxicity," *Journal of the American Medical Association,* Vol. 231 (1975), p. 1073.

Vitamin A (Retinol)

1. National Nutrition Consortium, Inc., *Vitamin-Mineral Safety, Toxicity, and Misuse* (Chicago: The American Dietetic Association, 1978).
2. Food and Drug Administration, "Vitamin and Mineral Drug Products for Over-the-Counter Human Use," *Federal Register*, Vol. 44 (March 16, 1979), pp. 16126-16201 (Vitamin A: pp. 16162-16164).
3. Adelle Davis, *Let's Eat Right to Keep Fit* (New York: Harcourt Brace Jovanovich, Inc., 1970).

Vitamin D

1. Food and Drug Administration, "Vitamin and Mineral Drug Products for Over-the-Counter Human Use," *Federal Register,* Vol. 44 (March 16, 1979), pp. 16126-16201 (Vitamin D: pp. 16164-16169).
2. Committee on Nutrition, The American Academy of Pediatrics, "The Prophylactic Requirement and the Toxicity of Vitamin D," *Pediatrics*, Vol. 31 (1963), pp. 512-525.
3. Catharyn Elwood, *Feel Like a Million* (New York: Pocket Books, 1965).
4. Adelle Davis, *Let's Eat Right to Keep Fit* (New York: Harcourt Brace Jovanovich, Inc., 1970).
5. E. Cheraskin, W.M. Ringsdorf Jr., and A. Brecher, *Psychodietetics: Food As the Key to Emotional Health* (New York: Stein and Day, 1974).
6. Food and Nutrition Board—National Research Council. *Recommended Dietary Allowances,* 8th ed. (Washington, D.C.: National Academy of Sciences, 1974).

Vitamin E (Tocopherol)

1. M.K. Horwitt, "Vitamin E in Human Nutrition—An Interpretive Review," *Borden's Review of Nutritional Research*, Vol. 22 (1961), p. 1.
2. M.K. Horwitt, "Vitamin E and Lipid Metabolism in Man," *American Journal of Clinical Nutrition*, Vol. 8 (1960), p. 451.

References

3. "Vitamin E, What's Behind All Those Claims for It?", *Consumer Reports*, Vol. 38 (January, 1973), pp. 60-66.
4. Adelle Davis, *Let's Eat Right to Keep Fit* (New York: Harcourt Brace Jovanovich, Inc., 1970).
5. A. Vogelsang and E.V. Shute, "Effect of Vitamin E in Coronary Heart Disease," *Nature*, Vol. 157 (1946), p. 772.
6. W.E. Shute, E.V. Shute, and A. Vogelsang, "Vitamin E in Heart Disease: the Anginal Syndrome," *Medical Record*, Vol. 160 (1947), p. 91.
7. W.E. Shute and H.J. Taub, *Vitamin E for Ailing and Healthy Hearts* (New York: Pyramid Books, 1972).
8. Catharyn Elwood, *Feel Like a Million* (New York: Pocket Books, 1965).
9. Richard A. Passwater, *Supernutrition—Megavitamin Revolution* (New York: Dial Press, 1975).
10. R.E. Gilliam, B. Mondell, and J.R. Warbasse, "Quantitative Evaluation of Vitamin E in the Treatment of Angina Pectoris," *American Heart Journal*, Vol. 93 (1977), p. 444.
11. Food and Drug Administration, "Vitamin and Mineral Drug Products for Over-the-Counter Human Use" *Federal Register*, Vol. 44 (March 16, 1979), pp. 16126-16201 (Vitamin E: pp. 16169-16173).
12. "Vitamin E—Miracle or Myth?" *FDA Consumer* (July-August, 1973), pp. 24-25.

Megavitamin Therapy

1. Richard A. Passwater, *Supernutrition—Megavitamin Revolution* (New York: Pocket Books, 1976), pp. 183-184.
2. Food and Nutrition Board-National Research Council, *Recommended Dietary Allowances*, 8th ed. (Washington, D.C.: National Academy of Sciences, 1974), pp. 2-3.
3. Food and Drug Administration, "Vitamin and Mineral Drug Products for Over-the-Counter Human Use," *Federal Register*, Vol. 44 (March 16, 1979), pp. 16126-16201.
4. E. Cheraskin and W.M. Ringsdorf Jr., *New Hope for Incurable Diseases* (Jericho, New York: Exposition Press, 1971).
5. C.E. Butterworth, "Review of New Hope for Incurable Diseases," *Journal of Nutrition Education*, Vol. 4 (1972), p. 181.
6. Adelle Davis, *Let's Eat Right to Keep Fit* (New York: Harcourt Brace Jovanovich, Inc., 1970).
7. S. Valsrub, "Editorial—Vitamin Abuse," *Journal of the American Medical Association*, Vol. 238 (1977), p. 1762.

Index

A

Abdec Kapseals multivitamin, 221
Abdol with Minerals multivitamin, 221
Abdec Baby Drops multivitamin, 220
absorption, 263
acne, 143
ACP (acyl carrier protein), 81
acrodermatitis enteropathica, 210
Adabee multivitamin, 222
Adabee with Minerals multivitamin, 223
Addison's disease, 78, 82
alcoholism, 201
Allbee multivitamin, 223
alpha-tocopherol, 161
  See also vitamin E
alpha-tocopherol acetate, 161
aluminum, 199

American Medical Association, 128
American Psychiatric Association, 69
amino acids, 263
anemia, 82, 102, 104, 106, 115, 164, 177, 188, 204, 206, 263
angina pectoris, 167
antagonist, 263
antihemorrhagic factor, 170
antioxidant, 263
antipernicious anemia factor, 112
antirachitic, 263
antiscorbutic, 263
antivitamin, 263
apoenzyme, 28, 263
ariboflavinosis, 54
arteriosclerosis, 263
arthritis, 78, 82, 157
ascorbic acid
  See vitamin C
atherosclerosis, 126, 264

Index

avidin, 98, 264

B

Basic Four Food Groups, 13, 14, 180, 264
beriberi, 39, 40, 42, 43, 176, 264
beta-tocopherol, 161
  See also vitamin E
bile, 264
bioflavonoids, 37
biotin, 26, 96-100, 264
  claims and controversy, 99
  CONSUMER GUIDE® magazine opinion of, 100
  deficiency of, 98
  dietary requirements for, 97
  food sources of, 97
  function of, 97
  hazards and toxicity of, 99
  history of, 96
  summary of, 100
  therapeutic uses of, 98
blood plasma, 264
blood serum, 264
Booher, L.E., 53
boron, 199
brand-name vitamin supplements, 219-262
Butterworth, C.E., 197

C

cadmium, 199
calcium, 20, 155, 156, 188, 199, 200-201, 210, 211
  sources of, 15
calorie, 10, 264
cancer, 105
carbohydrates, 10, 11, 20, 26, 27, 264
cardiac arrhythmias, 69
carotene, 138, 264
Cartier, Jacques, 121
Castle, William, 112
catalyst, 264
cataracts, 56
cheilosis, 264
Cheraskin, E., 196
chloride, 20, 201, 210

Chocks multivitamin (regular and Bugs Bunny), 224
Chocks Plus Iron multivitamin (regular and Bugs Bunny Plus Iron), 224
cholecalciferol, 264
cholesterol, 34, 264
choline, 36, 37, 186
chlorine, 199
chromium, 20, 199, 214
Clark, Linda, 82
coagulation Factor II, 171, 172, 173
coal tar, 30
cobalt, 20, 199, 203-204
cod liver oil, 153, 157
Cod Liver Oil Concentrate multivitamin, 225
coenzymes, 28, 264
collagen, 264
Combex Kapseals with Vitamin C multivitamin, 226
common cold, 120
compound, 264
connective tissue, 264
consumer product labeling, 16
copper, 20, 199, 204
Coronary Drug Project Research Group, 68
cyanocobalamin
  See vitamin B_{12}

D

Daily Food Guide, 14
Dam, Henrik, 170
Davis, Adelle, 36, 37, 56, 82, 91, 116, 143, 158, 166, 197
Dayalets multivitamin, 226
Dayalets plus Iron multivitamin, 226
deficiency, 264
delirium, 264
delta-tocopherol, 161
  See also vitamin E
deoxyribonucleic acid (DNA), 104, 105, 114, 115, 265
dermatitis, 264
Di-Cal D multivitamin, 227
diet
  purified, 264

Index

mixed, 265
digestion, 265
DNA
   See deoxyribonucleic acid

E

eczema, 37
Eijkman, Christiaan, 40
element, 265
Elvehjem, Conrad, 66
Elwood, Catharyn, 157, 167
enzyme, 28, 265
enrichment, 265
epithelium, 265
ergosterol, 153
essential amino acids, 20, 265
essential nutrients, 11, 265
   classes of, 20

F

fats, 10, 11, 20, 26, 27, 265
fatty acids, 265
FDA
   See Food and Drug
     Administration
Federal Register, 35
Feel Like a Million, 157, 167
Femiron iron supplement, 227
Femiron multivitamin, 228
Feosol iron supplement, 228
Fer-In-Sol iron supplement, 230
ferrous gluconate, 207
fetus, 265
Flintstones multivitamin, 230
Flintstones Plus Iron multivitamin, 231
fluorine, 20, 199, 204-205
folacin, 102-110, 265
   claims and controversy, 107
   CONSUMER GUIDE® magazine opinion of, 107
   content of common foods, 109-110
   deficiency of, 104
   dietary requirements for, 103
   food sources of, 103
   function of, 104
   hazards of, 106
   history of, 102
   summary of, 108
   therapeutic uses of, 106
folate
   See folacin
folic acid, 103, 117
Food and Drug Administration, 35, 68, 168, 173, 193, 194, 265
Food and Drug Administration Advisory Panel on Vitamin and Mineral Drug Products for Over-the-Counter Human Use, 44, 91, 98, 99, 106, 126, 143, 156, 195, 211
Food and Nutrition Board of the National Academy of Sciences, National Research Council, 12, 13, 41, 66, 87, 88, 103, 104, 123, 139, 184, 194, 265
fortification, 265
Four Food Group Plan, 14, 15, 16
Four Food Groups, 265
fructose, 265
Funk, Casimir, 26

G

gamma-tocopherol, 161
   See also vitamin E
Geritol Junior multivitamin (liquid), 231
Geritol Junior multivitamin (tablet), 232
Geritol multivitamin (liquid), 233
Geritol multivitamin (tablet), 234
Gevrabon multivitamin, 234
gluconeogenesis, 98
glucose, 265
glycogen, 265
Goldberger, Joseph, 65
Grijns, Gerrit, 40
Gyorgy, Paul, 97

H

hay fever, 37
Health and Nutrition Examination Survey (HANES), 177, 178
heart disease, 64
hemoglobin, 266

Index

hemorrhage, 266
hepatitis, 142
Herbert, Victor, 117
hesperidin, 37
Hippocrates, 31
Hopkins, Sir Frederick G., 25
hormones, 266
hydrochloric acid, 201
hydrogen chloride, 201
hyperthyroidism, 205
hypervitaminosis, 266
hypothyroidism, 205

I

Iberet-500 multivitamin (oral solution), 235
Iberet-500 multivitamin (tablet), 237
Iberet multivitamin (oral solution), 236
Iberet multivitamin (tablet), 237
Iberol multivitamin, 238
ileitis, 115
ileum, 266
Incremin with Iron multivitamin, 239
inositol, 36, 37
insulin, 209
intake, 266
intermittent claudication, 165
internal unit, 266
intrinsic factor, 111, 115, 116, 266
iodine, 20, 199, 205
iron, 15, 17, 20, 177, 188, 199, 204, 205-207
Ironized Yeast iron supplement, 239
isolate, 266
isoniazid, 90

K

kidney disease, 37, 201
kidney stones, 89
King, C.G., 122

L

laetrile, 37
Lavoisier, Antoine, 9

Leiner's disease, 99
Let's Eat Right To Keep Fit, 36, 56, 116
levodopa, 91
Lind, James, 31, 121
Linda Clark's Handbook of Natural Remedies for Common Ailments, 37
lipids, 266
lipoic acid, 37
Livitamin multivitamin (capsule), 240
Livitamin multivitamin (chewable tablet), 240
Livitamin multivitamin (liquid), 241

M

macrocytic anemia, 266
macroelement, 266
malabsorption, 266
magnesium, 20, 188, 199, 201-202
malaria, 105
manganese, 20, 199, 207-208
megadose, 266
megaloblastic anemia, 266
megavitamin therapy, 34, 266
menstruation, 15
metabolism, 10, 266
microcytic anemia, 266
microelement, 266
microorganisms, 266
minerals, 20, 198-218
  table of adult RDAs, food sources, and deficiency states, 198
mineral supplements, 187
Mol-Iron iron supplement, 242
molybdenum, 20, 199, 208
Monster Brand multivitamin, 243
mucosa, 266
Multicebrin multivitamin, 244
multivitamin, 266
muscular dystrophy, 166
Myadec multivitamin, 245
myelin, 114, 115
myopia, 158

N

National Center for Health

Index

Statistics, 177
natural vitamin supplements, 190-191
nausea, 266
nephritis, 37
New York State Court of Appeals, 193
New Hope for Incurable Diseases, 196
niacin, 64-71, 266
   claims and controversy, 68
   CONSUMER GUIDE® magazine opinion of, 69-70
   content of common foods, 72-73
   content in two typical daily diets, 76-77
   deficiency of, 67
   dietary requirements for, 66
   food sources of, 66
   function of, 67
   good sources of, 74-75
   hazards and toxicity of, 68
   history of, 65
   summary of, 70-71
   therapeutic uses of, 68
niacinamide, 267
nickel, 199
nicotinamide, 67, 68, 70
nicotinic acid, 34, 66, 67, 267
night blindness, 140, 141, 267
nonvitamins, 36
nutrient, 267
nutrition, 8-24, 267
   definition of, 8
   history of, 9
Nutrition Against Disease, 107
Nutrition Information panel, 16
   sample of, 18
Nutrition Program of the United States Public Health Service, 177
nyctalopia, 267

O

One-A-Day multivitamin, 245
One-A-Day multivitamin plus iron, 246
One-A-Day multivitamin plus minerals, 246

Optilets-500 multivitamin, 247
Optilets-M-500 multivitamin, 248
orthomolecular therapy, 34
osteomalacia, 155, 156, 267
OTC, 267
overage, 267
overdose, 267
oxalic acid, 89
oxidation, 267

P

PABA (p-aminobenzoic acid), 36, 37
Paladac multivitamin, 249
Paladac with Minerals multivitamin, 249
pangamic acid, 37
pantothenic acid, 78-86, 267
   claims and controversy, 71
   CONSUMER GUIDE® magazine opinion of, 82
   content of common foods, 84
   deficiency of, 81
   dietary requirements for, 80
   food sources of, 80
   function of, 81
   hazards and toxicity, 81
   history of, 79
   summary of, 82
   therapeutic uses of, 71
parasitic diseases, 37
Parkinson's disease, 91, 208
Passwater, Richard, 82, 99, 106, 126, 167, 193, 194, 195, 196
Pasteur, Louis, 32
Pauling, Linus, 120, 127
pellagra, 65, 66, 176, 267
penicillamine, 90
peptic ulcers, 68
pernicious anemia, 267
phosphorus, 20, 156, 188, 199, 200-201
plasma, 267
poison ivy, 37
poison oak, 37
polyneuritis, 267
polyunsaturated fatty acids, 124, 267
Poly-Vi-Sol multivitamin, 250

Index

Poly-Vi-Sol with Iron multivitamin, 251
potassium, 20, 199, 201, 202-203, 205, 210
proteins, 10, 11, 20, 26, 27, 267
   sources of, 14
Prout, William, 11
provitamin, 267
provitamin A, 29
provitamin D, 29
psoriasis, 105
Psychodietitics, 69, 107, 126, 158
pyridoxal, 87
pyridoxamine, 87
pyridoxine
   See vitamin B_6

R

rachitic rosary, 155
rancid, 268
RDA, 12, 267
   See also Recommended Dietary Allowances
Recommended Dietary Allowances, 12, 17
   See also listings and discussions under individual vitamins
   table of, 21-23
retinal, 268
retinol
   See vitamin A
rheumatic fever, 142
riboflavin (vitamin B_2), 27, 52-63, 87, 177, 268
   claims and controversy, 56
   CONSUMER GUIDE® magazine opinion of, 56
   content of common foods, 58-59
   content in two typical daily diets, 62-63
   deficiency of, 54-55
   dietary requirements of, 54
   food sources of, 53
   function of, 54
   good sources of, 60-61
   hazards and toxicity of, 55
   history of, 52
   summary of, 57
   therapeutic uses of, 55
ribonucleic acid (RNA), 209
rickets, 152, 156, 176, 200, 268
Ringsdorf, W.M., Jr., 196
RNA
   See ribonucleic acid
Rocky Mountain spotted fever, 37
rutin, 37

S

schizophrenia, 64, 69, 126, 192
Scott, Robert, 121
scurvy, 4, 31, 121, 124, 125, 176, 268
selenium, 20, 164, 199, 208-209
serum, 268
Shute, Evan, 166
Shute, Wilfred, 166
silicon, 199
Simron iron supplement, 251
sodium, 20, 199, 201, 203, 205, 210
staminal principles, 11
starch, 20
Stresscaps multivitamin, 252
Stresstabs 600 multivitamin, 252
Stuart Prenatal multivitamin, 253
subclinical deficiency, 268
Supernutrition—Megavitamin Revolution, 69, 99, 167
Super Plenamins multivitamin, 253
supplement, 268
symptom, 268
syndrome, 268
synthesis, 268
synthetic vitamins, 186
Szent-Gyorgyi, Albert, 122

T

Takaki, K., 40
Taub, Harold, 167
Ten State Nutrition Survey (TSNS), 176, 177, 178
Thera-Combex H-P multivitamin, 254
Theragran multivitamin (liquid), 254
Theragran multivitamin (tablet), 255

Index

Theragran-M multivitamin, 256
therapeutic, 268
thiamin (vitamin B$_1$), 17, 26, 29, 32, 39-51, 87, 177, 268
  claims and controversy, 44
  CONSUMER GUIDE® magazine opinion of, 44
  content of common foods, 46-47
  content in two typical daily diets, 48-49
  deficiency of, 42
  dietary requirements for, 41
  food sources of, 41
  function of, 42
  good sources of, 50-51
  hazards and toxicity of, 43
  history of, 40
  summary of, 44-45
  therapeutic uses of, 43
thrombosis, 126
thyroid hormones, 205
thyroxine, 205
tin, 199
tocopherol
  See vitamin E
toxicity, 268
transketolase, 32
triiodothyronine, 205
Tri-Vi-Sol multivitamin, 257
Tri-Vi-Sol with Iron multivitamin, 257
tryptophan, 89, 268
tyrosine, 205
tuberculosis, 90
typhus, 37

U

ultraviolet rays, 268
Unicap multivitamin (capsule), 258
Unicap multivitamin (chewable tablet; tablet), 258
Unicap M multivitamin, 259
Unicap Therapeutic multivitamin, 259
United States Department of Agriculture, 14
United States Recommended Daily Allowances, 16, 268
U.S. RDAs
  See United States Recommended Daily Allowances
U.S. RDA for Adults and Children over Four
  table of, 24

V

Valsrub, Samuel, 197
vanadium, 199
vascular, 268
Vi-Penta Infant Drops multivitamin, 260
Vi-Penta multivitamin, 261
visual purple, 268
vitamin, 268
vitamin A (retinol), 18, 26, 27, 29, 33, 124, 138-151, 177, 181, 182, 193
  claims and controversy, 143
  CONSUMER GUIDE® magazine opinion of, 143
  content of common foods, 145-146
  content in two typical daily diets, 151
  deficiency of, 141
  dietary requirements for, 139
  food sources of, 139
  function of, 140
  good sources of, 147-149
  hazards and toxicity of, 142
  history of, 138
  summary of, 144
  therapeutic uses of, 141
vitamin activity, 268
vitamin B$_1$
  See thiamin
vitamin B$_2$
  See riboflavin
vitamin B$_3$, 269
vitamin B$_5$, 269
vitamin B$_6$ (pyridoxine), 27, 30, 86-95
  claims and controversy, 91
  CONSUMER GUIDE® magazine opinion of, 91

Index

content of common food, 94-95
deficiency of, 89
dietary requirements for, 88
food sources of, 87
function of, 88
hazards and toxicity of, 90
history of, 86
summary of, 92
therapeutic uses of, 90
vitamin B$_{12}$ (cyanocobalamin), 11, 29, 102, 104, 111-119, 204
  claims and controversy, 116
  CONSUMER GUIDE® magazine opinion of, 117
  content of common food, 119
  deficiency of, 114
  dietary requirements for, 113
  food sources of, 113
  functions of, 114
  hazards and toxicity of, 116
  history of, 112
  summary of, 117-118
  therapeutic uses of, 115
vitamin B$_{15}$, 37, 269
vitamin B$_{17}$, 37, 269
vitamin C (ascorbic acid), 4, 17, 18, 26, 27, 31, 34, 120-137, 177, 181, 182, 192
  claims and controversy, 126
  CONSUMER GUIDE® magazine opinion of, 128
  content of common foods, 131-132
  deficiency of, 124
  dietary requirements for, 123
  food sources of, 122
  function of, 124
  good sources of, 133-137
  hazards and toxicity of, 125
  history of, 121
  summary of, 122
  therapeutic uses of, 125
Vitamin C and the Common Cold, 120, 126
vitamin content, 269
vitamin D, 26, 27, 33, 152-159, 165, 181, 182, 200
  claims and controversy, 157
  CONSUMER GUIDE® magazine opinion of, 158

  deficiency of, 155
  dietary requirements for, 154
  food sources of, 154
  function of, 155
  hazards and toxicity of, 156
  history of, 153
  summary of, 159
  therapeutic uses of, 155-156
vitamin D$_2$, 153
vitamin derivative, 269
vitamin E (tocopherol), 5, 27, 30, 33, 34, 124, 160-169, 184, 192, 268
  claims and controversy, 165
  CONSUMER GUIDE® magazine opinion of, 168
  deficiency of, 163
  dietary requirements for, 162
  food sources of, 162
  function of, 163
  hazards and toxicity of, 165
  history of, 161
  medical consensus of, 168
  summary of, 168
  therapeutic uses of, 165
Vitamin E for Ailing and Healthy Hearts, 167
vitamin F, 269
Vitamin H, 97
vitamin K, 26, 27, 33, 165
  CONSUMER GUIDE® magazine opinion of, 173
  deficiency of, 171
  dietary requirements for, 171
  food sources of, 171
  function of, 171
  hazards and toxicity of, 173
  history of, 170
  summary of, 173-174
  therapeutic uses of, 172
vitamin K$_1$, 171, 173
vitamin K$_2$, 171, 173
vitamin K$_3$, 171, 173
vitamin P, 269
vitamin potency, 269
vitamin Q, 269
vitamins, 19, 20
  discovery of, 11
  sources of, 14
  history of, 26

Index

identification of, 26
function of, 27
special needs for, 29
natural vs. synthetic, 30
toxicity, 33
megadoses, 33
therapeutic use, 33
vitamin supplements, 34 175-191
  and dieting, 180
  and eating habits, 181
  and pregnancy, 180
  and the elderly, 180
  composition of selected "natural" vitamin supplements, 190-191
  how to buy, 187
  individual product profiles, 219-262
  labeling of, 182-187
  need for, 178
vitamin U, 269
Vogelsang, Albert, 166

W

water-soluble vitamins, 27
Waugh, W.A., 122
Williams, Robert, 40
Williams, Roger, 82, 107
Wills, Lucy, 102
Windmill Natural Vitamin Company, 37

X

xanthurenic acid, 89
xerophthalmia, 141, 269

Z

zinc, 20, 188, 199, 209-210, 211
Zymalixir multivitamin, 261
Zymasyrup multivitamin, 262

FUNDERBURG LIBRARY
MANCHESTER COLLEGE

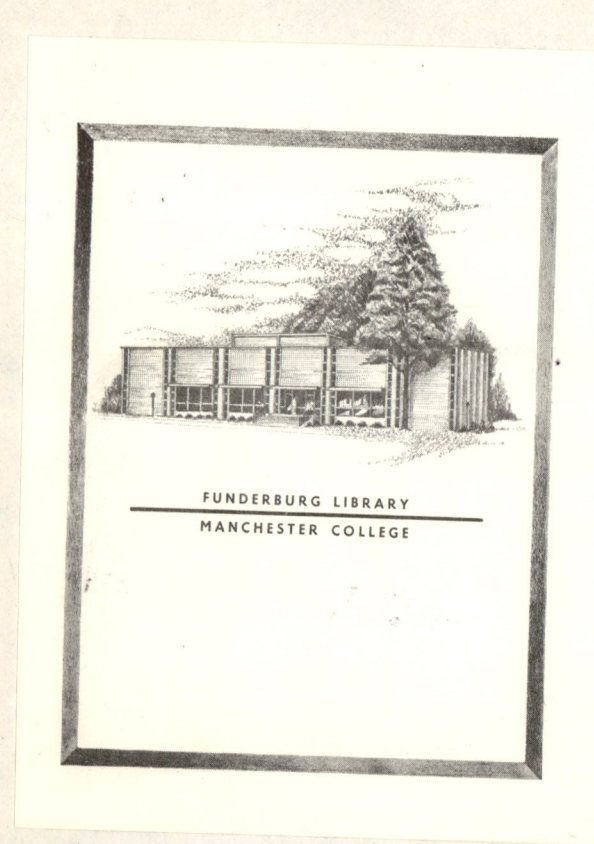